30 days Microbiome Anti-Diet

Relaxed - healthy nutrition
for individualists

Katrin Zahnweh

Contents

Preface

Anyone interested in the Microbiome Anti-Diet has a clear goal: health, well-being and... down with the gastrointestinal problems!

A conversation between friends, colleagues or relatives rarely takes this direction. To the classic small talk opening "How are you?" hardly anyone answers "Oh, not so good, my bowels are causing problems!". But as soon as we start talking - more or less bashfully - about our own gastrointestinal problems, we quickly find out that an incredible number of people in our own environment are also affected. From slight pinching and embarrassing flatulence to constant pain that makes life hell, there is just about everything. Healthy people (and pretty much all men) usually eat relatively carefree and worry little about what is happening inside the body. Somehow this body does it all by itself... But only very few (enviable) people have this condition for a lifetime. Many of us sooner or later realize with concern that something is not quite right with our digestion or general state of health.

At the latest then we fall into actionism and want to do something good for our intestines and the army of microbes that live in them. But then the next problem arises. What exactly should this "good thing" look like? Advertising and media flood us daily with ever new nutritional trends. One day they promote something as insanely healthy, just one week later the same thing is incredibly harmful or near to fatal.

The Food Combining Diet has been running for just two weeks, but suddenly all the magazines and news portals are warning against animal fat, which rather contradicts the Food Combining Diet. But don't worry. Food Combining is for sissies anyway. The modern Homo Sapiens must be at least vegan, go through one detox cure after the other or meticulously avoid any trace of carbohydrates if he still wants to be hip. Best of all, all at once, a carbohydrate-free vegan detox diet. The dietary victim can endure extreme dietary changes of any kind, depending on his personal tolerance for suffering, for between one and six months, before he throws in the towel and shouts "F*** the healthy diet! "

But it is also damned complicated to choose one from the mass of nutritional forms. How are we supposed to know what the "right" nutrition is, and is nutrition alone even sufficient to support the intestines and be healthy? The desperate search for the holy grail of nutrition sooner or later leads the tormented diet victim to various websites. Finally, the solution is in sight! In addition to information on the subject of health, various miracle cures are offered there, which should cure practically any illness in no time, from ingrown toenails to pancreatic cancer. For only twenty euros per thirty milliliters. When something is that expensive, the effect must be immense, right? Click-click-click, and your virtual shopping basket is already full of grapefruit seed extract, base capsules, yacon powder, various minerals and the big 4-week detox treatment. If the hoped-for effect does not occur after taking the product, it must be our fault. Surely, we have forgotten to take one of the five portions of tablets, capsules and drops prescribed daily during the last week or have done something else wrong.

If the miracle cures fail, there is only one thing left: Now we are going radical! A bowel cleansing, or better yet a complete bowel rehabilitation, is needed. As the perfect introduction to the diet, we choke down a kind of cat litter in capsule or powder form to cleanse the intestines and swallow a handful of algae tablets to absorb valuable nutrients - the same nutrients that were swept away a few minutes earlier during the cleanse. We take capsules with bacteria, only to flush them out again during the daily colon hydrotherapy (that's the thing with water up the ass... sorry, into the *colon*). After all, we have to get rid of all those weird and nasty deposits that accumulate in our intestines over the course of our lives.

If you could smile or nod your head a few times while reading and have had enough of miracle cures and extremism in the area of nutrition and health for a long time, this is the place to be. All this can be done more easily. Healthier. Cheaper. And more pleasant.

Anti-Diet?

Why is the Anti-Diet the better solution? No matter what new diet you are on, it usually begins as follows: The delinquent chooses a period of time when there are no temptations that could lead to a break in the diet. Holidays, birthdays, holidays, celebrations and other sources of temptation must therefore be carefully avoided. Somewhere in the calendar two or three perfect weeks without special events have finally found each other and the ordeal can begin.

The Standard Diet

Finally, the right diet has been found. Eight pounds less in two weeks, doesn't that sound marvelous? After that, everything will finally be different, and our new, healthier life will begin. In preparation, the refrigerator, kitchen cabinets and pantry are critically examined and food worth several hundred euros is disposed of - after all, all that unhealthy stuff is to be avoided in the future. Then we go shopping full of enthusiasm and order the craziest stuff online. Things that our grandma has never heard of before. We spend a lot of money on miso paste, tempeh, goji berries and acai powder and only find out how expensive all this fun was when we receive our next credit card bill. The next step leads us to the local grocery stores, where we stock up with mountains of fresh fruits and vegetables. With a mixture of superiority and envy we look at the shopping of the person in front, who is just paying for frozen pizza, chocolate and cheeseballs. Then the diet begins.

Diary of a Diet Victim

Day 1: I am highly motivated! The whole kitchen is full of healthy stuff. It's nice. My friends already know that I will soon weigh 20 pounds less and live healthier from now on. Anyway, the dinner wasn't that bad today!

Day 2: Today we had rice, a welcome change from the low-fat cabbage soup of yesterday. I had to get up an hour earlier in the morning to have breakfast and prepare my lunch for the office, but I'm worth it.

Day 3: Today the food was delicious again. I only needed one teaspoon of the miso paste for the soup. Unfortunately, the paste was only available in block format. Well, then there is miso soup from time to time, it tastes not bad.

Day 4: Presentation to the management at nine o'clock in the morning, and the slides were not yet ready. So, breakfast was far too stressful for me today. I ate twice as much at lunchtime, so it will be fine. After work I had to go shopping. It's a little stressful...

Day 5: I already feel incredibly light, I think the diet is working! It's not easy, but everything's hard at the beginning - I follow through!

Day six: "Watch TV in the evening and nibble on carrot strips instead of chocolate." Who gives that kind of advice? Well, the things you do...

Day 7: This morning I simply did not manage to prepare lunch. Nevertheless, I was really hungry. So, I sinned. On the other hand, a single curry sausage is certainly not important. But I still have a guilty conscience, actually I wanted to stick to the guidelines one hundred percent.

Day 8: Zucchini? I actually can't stand them, but according to the diet plan there are stuffed zucchini today. Well, they'll be good for something. Uh...

Day 9: Whew. The vegetable remains pile up in the refrigerator. What do I do with all this stuff now? Today I have to take inventory and dispose of some stuff. Too bad for the money and expensive food.

Day 10: Where the heck am I supposed to get yellowfin tuna fillets in sushi quality in Pinckney, Michigan? What are these dietary inventors thinking?

Day 11: Hum, at the beginning I lost a lot of weight and felt completely detoxified, but now not a single gram goes down. Although I am hungry all the time. My boyfriend and my colleagues are also so obnoxious at the moment!

Day 12: Today I simply didn't have the strength for sports and had to give up. I want to watch TV and eat choco-laaaaaate! On top of that I had to cancel an invitation to-day. I would have loved to go, but how am I supposed to keep up my diet?

Day 13: Eda... WHAT... should I buy??? Edamame? What's that? I wonder if Albertsons has it.

Day 14: Enough. I can't see any more vegetables. And cer-tainly not raw or steamed. Thank God the diet is over, six pounds down. Now I take a break and try to lose another six pounds later.

Month two after the diet: Damn. I put back the six pounds, and I put another one on top. But no one can live on these steamed vegetables, and who can afford all these ingredi-ents in the long run? Well, actually I'm not that fat com-pared to my other friends... Am I making burgers or mac and cheese today?

3 years after the diet: Today I discovered something strange in a corner of the kitchen cupboard: An almost full, but completely dried up package of

"miso paste". How does that stuff get there?

It really doesn't have to be this way. It can also be more relaxed, cheaper and without wasting food. But with the help of a few trillion new friends, the microbiome. And with the Anti-Diet.

The Anti-Diet

Let's be honest - we've already tried it all, mostly with dubious results: diets, cures, and lately "challenges" (synonym for torture and renunciation). We've had enough of these diets and simply want to know how we can live a relaxed life without bending over backwards every day. The Microbiome-Anti-Diet leads us there step by step. With a lot of background knowledge and a guide for individualists who don't want endless shopping lists and detailed diet plans. This book is intended to inspire you to go your own way, which best suits your personal lifestyle: Relaxed and microbiome-friendly nutrition for individualists.

The tips do not come from a celebrity or fitness guru with a lot of time and money, a personal trainer on his side, and a body that has always been flawless and fat-free. Instead, they are based on the experiences of an absolute average person who has lived through all the ups and downs of health, nutrition, sports, dream figure and constant stress for several decades and is constantly learning. The tips for individualists help to support the microbiome, intestines and immune system - without the need for diets or extreme cures. Hence the name "Anti-Diet".

It is precisely because the Anti-Diet is so relaxed that it is not only suitable for 30 days, but for a whole life. To get started, however, it is easier to set a time-limited goal - "a lifetime" simply sounds too final. 30 days, on the other hand, are quite manageable. The tips can be applied very flexibly, depending on your own preferences. If inspiration is lacking at the beginning, it is still not easy to just get started. That's why the Anti-Diet provides suggestions and shows that a microbiome-friendly lifestyle is possible without a lot of effort and sacrifice. With the concentrated knowledge about our microbial friends and some inspiration through a few concrete examples, it is not at all difficult to support the microbiome and improve personal health. And all this without cat litter, I promise!

The Microbiome

The microbiome is the new intestinal flora, and it is part of our body and our Anti-Diet. It's hip, it's incredibly interesting, science is working on it fiercely, and the results are more than promising. If you put all the intestinal bacteria on the scale, they would weigh two to four pounds. Thanks to its numerous functions, the microbiome is even called an independent organ.

Goodbye Gut Flora - Hello Microbiome!

The designation "gut flora" or "intestinal flora" is actually already somewhat outdated. It comes from a time when the microscope and, with its help, the tiny creatures that colonize humans were only just discovered. These creatures were initially mistaken for plants (flora). When dealing with microscopically small dots and sticks, such a mix-up can happen... Their community in our colon was therefore unceremoniously called intestinal flora. The name is still familiar to most people today. It has been kind of tolerated for decades, although bacteria and other unicellular organisms are neither animals nor plants, but microorganisms.

For some years now, however, these microorganisms have been gaining prestige, making every B-lister green with envy. When the human genome was decoded, the result was quite disappointing and somehow embarrassing. Even very small and simple creatures such as mice or cucumber plants have approximately the same number of genes as humans. The crown of creation must first digest this unexpected result. The success of the project came, however, only a little later. This happens quite often in science, especially in medicine. In this case, the methods of gene sequencing had improved so much during the long-term project that a genome can now be decoded within a very short time. After the analysis of humans, science therefore set out to study even the smallest living creatures, our microorganisms.

This project produced one of the most astonishing results of the last decades: every human being is colonized by trillions of bacteria, no matter how thoroughly they wash their hands. Most of them live in the colon. If you don't constantly work with large numbers, you probably can't tell the number of zeros of a trillion right away without cheating (there are 12). No wonder, because we don't usually deal with such numbers in everyday life. Very convenient for politicians around the world who make themselves comfortable on a mountain of trillions of national debt, while we cannot even begin to imagine how much money this actually is and what this mountain of debt means for our future. But back to the population of bacteria inside us, where this large number is welcome and desirable, and to the genes.

If we had met an alien a few years ago and asked: "What are you?", we would have answered: "A human being". According to the latest scientific findings, the answer today would have to be: "A being consisting of one part human and several trillion parts microorganisms". This enormous amount of bacteria together have many more genes than its human counterparts. The exact numbers vary greatly in the various publications, but the factor ten is most frequently cited. Our brain first has to process this information before we can move on.

In the combination of microbiome and human, humans possess only ten percent of the genes! The remaining 90 percent come from the microorganisms on and in our body! There are also critical voices about this figure. It is sometimes said to be a calculation error, because this figure was deduced from the extreme density of bacteria in the colon, although it does not apply to the entire body. Unfortunately we cannot recount to find out the truth. But it doesn't make much difference whether it is actually 90 percent of genes and cells or a little less. One thing is certain: there are an incredible number. But science has found out a lot more. This enormous amount of microorganisms including their genes does not just live in and on us by chance and just bounce or crawl or float around senselessly, but our living together is vital - especially for us humans!

This groundbreaking insight helped the inner microbial community to make its big breakthrough in the public eye, including PR advice, a spruced-up image and a new, more dignified name, "microbiota". The **genes** of the microbiota are called microbiome. In the course of time, however, the term microbiome (which I think is a bit nicer) has become established for both. That is why I use it for the community of bacteria and not exclusively for their genes - may science forgive me.

The largest part of our microbiome is therefore located in our colon. Its wall is covered with them all over. A practical comparison gives a better feeling for the amount of microorganisms we are dealing with. In 2019, the earth was populated with about 7.6 billion people, moving around in 1.3 billion cars. A single gram of the contents of a colon is said to contain between 100 million and 10 billion microorganisms.

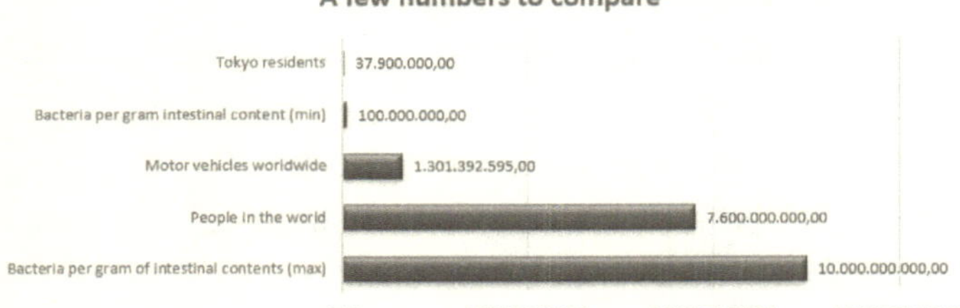

Relations: Bacteria per gram intestinal content and other numbers

Even in the minimum case, more bacteria live in a single gram of stool than people in Tokyo. In the maximum case it is even more than the entire world population.

A Young Friendship and Infinite Possibilities

Microbiome research is a very young field of science, it is, so to speak, only just hatching. The following two diagrams show how young this research is from a historical perspective.

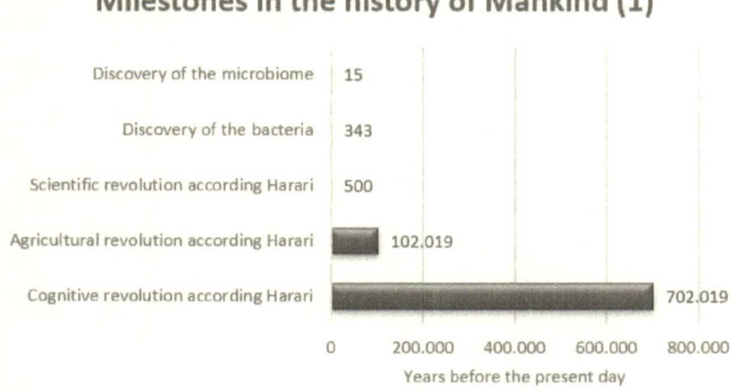

From the cognitive revolution to the discovery of the microbiome

According to the historian Harari, the cognitive revolution is the point in time from which Homo Sapiens developed the consciousness we have today. It was only from this point on that man was able to develop and spread abstract ideas, such as belief in spirits or gods [1]. Through this decisive cut, man could unite (or let himself be united) into larger groups with the help of ideologies and became the most dangerous predator on earth. The agricultural revolution, which transformed Homo Sapiens from a hunter to a farmer, came much later. The time in which we live today is marked by the scientific revolution, whose bars can hardly be seen in the first diagram, just like the discovery of bacteria and the microbiome. Therefore, the next diagram zooms in a little further into this area.

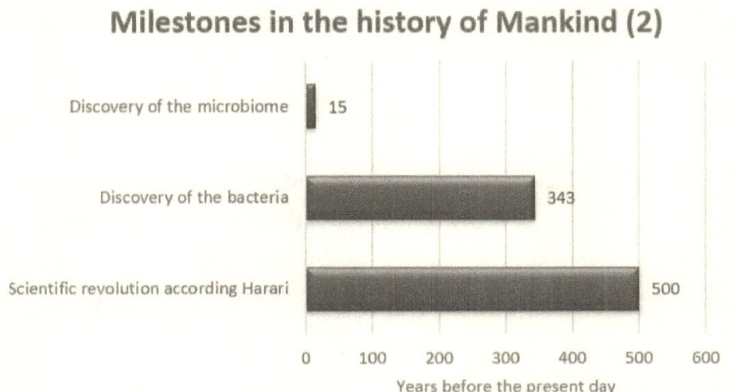

From the scientific revolution to the discovery of the microbiome

The second diagram shows even better how young the knowledge of our microbiome is compared to the total duration of the scientific era. This short detour makes it clear that we have only just begun to get to know our bacteria-friends better. However, it will still take some time before we really understand them - if humans and bacteria survive that long. A lot will happen until then. Some of what is considered safe today will certainly turn out to be a misconception in a few years' time.

The following applies to all scientific work: it costs money and must be financed. In principle, financial means also have financial interests behind them. Under these conditions, research results of all kinds and their publication in the mass media must generally be viewed critically. Not everything happens exclusively for the benefit of mankind. Pessimists like me would even claim that the welfare of mankind is probably at most just a random by-product. But sometimes the results of research actually benefit both sides. Everyone can benefit from it if he takes a closer look at the matter and draws the right conclusions for himself.

Microbiome research will certainly be aimed primarily at the creation of new products. If it is possible to offer a combination of bacteria in capsule form that makes us slim or cures chronic intestinal diseases, a nice chunk of money can be made. A patient with a long history of suffering will of course be happy to spend money on this modern medicine if it is proven to provide relief or cure. Therefore the sale and thus a certain profit are legitimate. However, we should by no means just rely on these modern products, but at the same time take advantage of the opportunities which nobody earns the big money with. These are not quite as easy to implement as the daily intake of a capsule and therefore continue to be a Cinderella subject. There are many ways to support our microbiome, starting with a critical and responsible use of antibiotics and a microbiome-friendly diet. Granted, this is not the "easy way for lazy people". The individualist needs a bit more knowledge, discipline and self-confidence to live in relaxed friendship with the microbes community.

Much remains to be explored. It is still unclear which composition a perfect microbiome should actually have, because there are so many different ones. The microbiome of a single person is said to be as unique as this person's fingerprint. If you consider that a fingerprint consists of a limited number of grooves in a rather small area, while the microbiome is composed of thousands of different species in varying numbers, it is quite obvious. The interaction of different species of bacteria with each other is still a great mystery, and this in a world that already believes to know everything. No one can yet say exactly what influence the microbiome has on the development of diseases of civilization, our actions and our thinking. But whatever the answer to these questions, it is certainly worthwhile to support our microbiome as much as possible. The best way to do this is to find out more about this fascinating creature. In the drawer "pretty sure" there are already some findings. If we take these into account, we are already quite well able to take care of our microbiome in an optimal way until science finds out more. This is exactly our goal.

Bad Guys & Good Cops

Even after several years, science is still at the very beginning of microbiome research. Until recently, bacteria were bad guys and had to be destroyed by antibiotics and disinfection. Since the great breakthrough of medically effective antibiotics, these bacteria killers have been perfected more and more. In addition to broad-spectrum antibiotics, antibiotics have been developed that act very specifically - a small step forward after all. Because there will always be situations in which it is not wise to do without antibiotics, despite all the bacterial friendship. Of course, these not only cause damage, but also have an undeniable benefit. Diseases caused by bacteria, which used to kill millions of people in agony, were eradicated virtually overnight and are no longer a threat today. The almost sterile life in the western world, starting at birth, also contributes to the decimation of bacterial infections.

But unfortunately there is a second side to the coin. Today it is becoming increasingly clear that man and environment are paying a very high price for this blanket destruction of all microbial life. Resistant bacteria are now one of the top ten threats to humanity. Allergies and diseases of civilization ensure that more and more people cannot enjoy life in full health. Bacteria are sometimes, but not always, the bad guys, and the unconditional fight against them can only be lost in the long run.

The bacteria in and around us are an important part of our own evolutionary history, and we cannot live without them, but only together with them. "Healthy with the microbiome" is therefore the motto. To do this, we must rethink, jettison some of our habits and adopt new ones. To live in friendship and super-healthy with the microbiome means to refrain from unnecessarily destroying bacteria and at the same time to support the bacteria that are useful to us as much as possible, especially through a bacteria-friendly nutrition. But nobody really wants to stick to a kind of lifelong weight-reduction plan and do without all the fun and pleasure in life. No problem, because it can be done quite differently. It is not only exciting, but also very useful to explore the symbiosis of the microbiome and the human body. Developing your own strategies that fit in with your personal life is then very easy. The cooperation between the human being and the microbiome is easier to understand if we start from scratch - with digestion.

The Miracle of … Digestion

The digestive system is a miracle, just like actually the whole body, there is no other way to say it. Sophisticated chemical and mechanical actions break down the apple we eat, without thinking much about it, into tiny little components that our body can absorb. The whole apple goes in - brownish-residue-about-what-we-do-not-talk-about-it comes out. But between "in" and "out" fascinating things happen!

Our organism cannot simply absorb and process apple pieces, no matter how devotedly we chew them. To absorb it, the apple, just like the piece of chocolate that may follow, must first be broken down into its smallest components, for example various nutrients, glucose and amino acids. These are so tiny that they can enter our bloodstream through the intestinal wall. But how does this work?

Digestion already begins in the mouth. That is why what responsible parents have always told their children applies: chewing thoroughly is very important. Firstly, because it shreds the food and the stomach must produce less acid to correct a sloppy job. On the other hand, because the food is mixed with saliva during chewing and the enzymes contained in it already predigest it. Starch, for example, can already be converted into sugar molecules in the mouth. This is why bread tastes slightly sweetish after long chewing.

The stomach itself starts to produce a digestive juice (not to be confused with the ever-popular digestive), which consists of enzymes and hydrochloric acid, long before this. These enzymes break down the absorbed proteins. Hydrochloric acid is classified as a hazardous material and irritates the skin, respiratory tract and eyes. In an open-body operation, you should actually find a large hazardous substance sticker on the stomach. If the stomach did not have its mucous membrane and, at the same time, cells with a high capacity for regeneration, it would actually digest itself by supplying hydrochloric acid. But as long as our stomach mucous membrane is intact, fortunately only the food that is in the stomach is dissolved.

In addition to this chemical dissolution, the stomach itself starts moving. Through strong contractions it kneads the chyme like granny kneads a yeast dough and pushes it towards the exit - into the duodenum. The porter makes sure that only tiny little pieces get into the intestine and not the slightly larger piece of apple that we swallowed in a hurry.

Of course, we don't usually eat apples only, but also much more substantial (and delicious) things, which usually contain more or less large amounts of fat. This doesn't bother our body as long as the quantity and quality is right. As soon as fatty food reaches the duodenum, the gallbladder and pancreas become active. The gallbladder releases the stored bile into the intestines to support the breakdown of fat.

Interesting to know: The gallbladder is just a storage location. It doesn't produce any bile. The liver does that instead. Once the gallbladder has been removed (cholecystectomy), people can only tolerate very little fat in their food. He can only make use of the amount of bile that can be produced by the liver on demand. Most of the bile is broken down again immediately "after use" or used by the microorganisms in the intestine. However, a small residue remains in the food pulp and colors it brownish - hence the color of the end product, which we all know. By means of a simple optical recognition procedure (scientifically speaking, it sounds much less disgusting), some diseases can also be detected at home. A very light-colored stool, for example, indicates problems with the liver or gall bladder. Problems with fat loss, such as nausea or colic after a high-fat meal, can indicate a disease of the gallbladder, such as gallstones. In such cases, it is important to shamelessly inform the family doctor about these embarrassing details and thus help him or her with the diagnosis.

The pancreas adds another important digestive juice. It neutralizes the hydrochloric acid from the stomach, which is a good idea for obvious reasons. In addition, due to its content of numerous, different enzymes, the digestive juice is able to break down practically everything into its components - with the exception of plant fibers (cellulose). But this is not a flaw in the system, because these plant fibers come into play a little later and perform an important task.

Now we head on to the next station, the small intestine. The chyme is mechanically moved further and further forward by the small intestine. There is no turning back, like in the queue before the roller coaster. Again enzymes are used to break down the remaining components of the food. Now these are so tiny that they penetrate through the wall of the intestine like through a very fine-meshed filter, and can then travel through the body in the bloodstream to their destination. The remaining food residues in the intestine contain almost no nutrients at this point and could actually be excreted even now. But there is another step towards the exit. In this step our main actors, the intestinal bacteria, finally come into play.

One of the tasks of the colon is to remove water and salts from the food pulp. From here on, the food chyme is pushed back and forth until the large intestine has fulfilled its tasks. From now on, the food pulp is called "stool", has become firmer and in the end always contains the same amount of salt. But this is not the only task of the large intestine. Probably the most important characteristic is that the large intestine is home to trillions of microorganisms which we share our lives with. We can make their existence pleasant or rather poor, and accordingly they too can benefit or harm us, depending on how well our intercultural cooperation works. The digestion process ends at this point, food remains and dead bacteria leave the body in the familiar way, and we mingle loosely with the microbial community to see what happens.

Bacteria as Digestive Aid

Herbivores produce the enzyme cellulase, which can effectively break down plant fibers (cellulose). Humans lack this enzyme, which is why plant fibers from our food migrate undigested into the large intestine. And this is where the feast for the intestinal microbiota, also called intestinal flora, begins. For it is precisely these plant fibers, which would be nothing but waste for ourselves, that are the preferred food for our bacteria.

However - and this is where it gets pretty scary - our intestinal bacteria also feed on our intestinal mucosa. Basically there is nothing wrong with this, because dead cells are removed by our bacteria in this way and can be replaced by new ones, a kind of free daily peeling. However, if the bacteria starve because they do not have enough fiber available, it becomes problematic. One study showed that the starving microbiota becomes aggressive and removes larger amounts of the intestinal mucosa than usual. Dr Mahesh Desai put it something like this: *"In other words, if you don't feed them, they can eat you."* [2].

Not only does this sound frightening, but it also has terrible consequences. The intestinal mucosa fulfils an important function, because through it the intestinal contents remain reliably in the intestine with no chance to escape to the outside. Microorganisms that are at home in our intestines really have no place in our bloodstream. Here they would cause great damage. Through a perforated intestinal wall, also called "leaky gut syndrome", microorganisms of all kinds, including pathogenic germs, can get into the blood. Not only the microorganisms themselves, but also their metabolic products slip through the intestinal mucosa in unusually high numbers, are distributed throughout the body via the bloodstream and can damage the nerve system.

The small intestine is another place where our bacteria are not welcome. If bacterial growth becomes excessive there, a problem called "bacterial overgrowth" develops, which can lead to painful bloating of the small intestine. This incorrect settlement is one of the many symptoms that are probably very often labelled with the very general diagnosis of "irritable bowel". There is a relatively harmless method to detect the small intestine malcolonization. The doctor can carry out a breath test to provide certainty. However, the subsequent treatment is somewhat more difficult and less harmless. In most cases, treatment with antibiotics is prescribed.

From a purely logical point of view (and my personal non-medical angle), this antibiotic treatment can actually only worsen the overall situation of the patient, even if many doctors apparently disagree. It might be that at the moment it is the only available method to provide short-term relief to the patient. However, there is a certain probability that the patient's intestinal problems will reappear after some time - in the worst case even reinforced, since not only the illegal settlers in the small intestine are killed, but also a large proportion of the bacteria in the large intestine that are vital for us. After that it is a matter of luck whether the good or an army of bad microbes first occupy the vacant positions.

Another reason for justified doubts about antibiotic therapy: The false colonization may be both symptom and cause at the same time. It is the cause of flatulence that plagues the patient, but could also be a symptom of a completely different problem, such as an unfavorable diet or a problem with the Bauhin valve, which prevents backflow from the large intestine into the small intestine. Neither of these can be eliminated by taking antibiotics.

Before taking antibiotics, it is definitely worth considering and trying out other options first - such as a time-limited gentle diet, a more conscious eating behavior, longer breaks between meals, lots of light exercise and little stress. In other words, anything that protects our microbiome and does not cause additional bloating, but at the same time reduces the food supply of the wild settlers in the small intestine somewhat and gives the intestine the chance to cleanse itself.

The Microbiome as Caretaker

The intestinal mucosa is one of the most important building blocks for our health and the seat of most immune cells. It consists of a dense network of epithelial cells, which can be imagined as small cobbles, with the mucus layer above. Although the latter sounds slippery and somewhat disgusting, together with the wall of epithelial cells it ensures that the contents of the intestine are encapsulated and cannot enter the abdominal cavity or the bloodstream - except by controlled transformation into usable nutrients.

This is where our microbes come in. They are anything but useless, let alone parasites. Bacteria not only colonize the intestines, but also look after their residential area extremely carefully, according to a similar principle to the renovation of a wooden garden house. First, old and loose parts of the wood have to be removed, then the new paint is applied as protection against the weather. Our bacteria eat the intestinal mucosa, thus ensuring a healthy peeling and stimulating the formation of new cells. At the same time some of our bacteria produce fatty acids, for example butanoic acid (butyric acid). This fulfils several important tasks at once. It serves the cells of the intestinal mucosa as an important source of energy, strengthens the connections between the epithelial cells (tight junctions) and counteracts inflammation.

The connection between inflammation, butyric acid and microbiome was investigated in a small study on Crohn's disease.

The diversity of different bacterial species was severely restricted in the microbiota of the patients. The amount of butyric acid in the intestine was also related to the degree of the disease - the lower the amount of butyric acid, the worse the degree of the disease. In such investigations, the question of cause and effect basically arises, but perhaps the answer is not so important for ourselves. There is a dependency, in this case a contrary course of inflammation and bacterial diversity including butyric acid production. Whatever the trigger - the only lever we have is the support of the microbes. We have no direct influence on anything else. In contrast to the intake of artificial anti-inflammatory drugs, microbe-friendly nutrition is a measure that certainly does not result in harmful side effects.

The microbial community, however, gives its people much more. Plant fibers that arrive in our large intestine provide an optimal volume of stool, but otherwise they do not bring any further benefits for humans. If it weren't for our friends, the bacteria. Not only do they eat these fibers, but they also metabolize them into essential vitamins and nutrients. This is again a very interesting insight. Our own vitamin supply depends not only on how many vitamins we take in with our food, but also on the vitamins produced by our microbiome.

Bouncers, Trainers and Squatters - The Microbiome and our Immune System

Our health depends to a very large extent on the functioning of our immune system. If the immune system goes crazy, for example by underreacting or overreacting, we have really lost. Either the immune system simply does not fend off harmful pathogens or it attacks everything highly aggressively, in the worst case even our own cells. The best way to support the immune system in its normal function is to strengthen the microbiome. We know now at the latest that bacteria eat food remnants that are indigestible for us, and that something is also coming out of the bacteria "behind". These are metabolic products, such as butyric acid, in technical jargon called "metabolites". The interaction between the immune system and the countless substances and micro-organisms that romp about in our body is absolutely fascinating. Therefore, we should definitely take a closer look at it.

Our immune system performs a very difficult task. It is our personal doorman and must detect and eliminate harmful intruders without delay and with one hundred percent certainty. In the classic first-person shooter (we are now moving in the world of nerds), it is very easy to lose your life in "friendly fire" if your fellow player cannot distinguish friend from foe in the hectic pace of the game. This must not happen to our immune system. It must distinguish between dangerous intruders, friendly bacteria and our own cells. Every mistake has a fatal effect on our health.

An example of such a defect of the immune system, also called autoimmune disease, is type 1 diabetes. In this disease, the patient's own immune system attacks the insulin-producing cells of the pancreas. To prevent such embarrassing and serious mistakes from happening, the immune system needs to be perfectly trained. This training takes place in the intestine. Why in the intestine of all places, and how does such training work?

For a good training you usually need enough space. This is guaranteed by the enormous size of the intestine, which is the result of a small but very cool trick of nature. We know the intestine as a long tube that somehow winds its way through our abdominal cavity, and it is relatively unspectacular. Or also as a natural packaging of sausages (somehow "ew!"). But through a clever combination of folds and the finest ramifications, the actual surface of the intestine is enormous. When unfolded, it should be about 400 to 500 square meters. The skin, on the other hand, only covers a measly 1.7 square meters on average. Quite impressive - unfortunately, I have not yet been able to personally measure it to confirm the truth of the 400 square meter statement. So let's believe it for now without checking.

But the intestine does not just have a large surface area and lies around lazily in our stomach. The crucial point is: The intestine is actually our largest contact surface to the outside world, even if it sounds absurd. Because everything we swallow in life ends up in the intestine - unless, after a drunken night, it goes in the opposite direction, but let's leave that alone. Through food and drink we bring the outside world into the intestines, so to speak. That's why it makes sense that a very large proportion of our immune cells are located directly in the intestinal mucosa (the figures given vary between 30 and 80 percent - perhaps someone should count a little more precisely). These immune cells are automatically confronted with everything we ingest. This includes not only nutrients, but also a colorful mix of useful bacteria, harmful pathogens and allergenic substances.

For this reason, the intestine is also the perfect place where the vital training of our immune cells can take place. Here they are prepared for their later function, with our good microbes as sparring partners and trainers. The cells are only released into the bloodstream when they have completed their training absolutely faultlessly. However, this training is one of the hardest in the world, there is no mercy and no second chance here. A small mistake of the immune cell inevitably leads to its destruction. In view of this, we might be quite happy about our own job choice after all. If, on the other hand, the immune cell reacts correctly, it passes the training. It identifies a certain component of the food pulp as harmful, for example listeria or salmonella. It then begins to form antibodies to render the intruder harmless. Immune cells activated in this way are now released into the bloodstream via the intestinal mucosa and spread throughout the body, where they continue to form antibodies against the harmful substance that is on their personal blacklist. However, there are other participants in the training, namely our bacteria friends.

What Joachim Löw is to the German national football team is our microbiome for the immune system. It not only has the function of a coach, but is also the chief strategist. The microbiome determines what kind of immune cells are produced and how aggressive or relaxed they react to intruders. Even the formation of our blood group is based on our microbiome. There is a very exciting paragraph about this in Julia Enders' book "Gut - The inside story of our body's most under-rated organ". A newborn baby, which does not yet have a significant intestinal flora and a mature immune system, could theoretically be given any blood group. Only when the microbiome is fully developed do the immune cells learn to regard foreign blood groups as hostile.

However, the multitasking capabilities of our microbiome are not yet exhausted. In addition to its tasks as bouncer, trainer and strategist, it is also a successful squatter. Simply by taking up space in the intestine, our beneficial bacteria already fend off unwanted invaders that have survived the bath in stomach acid. When the football stadium is one hundred percent occupied by peaceful fans, there are no more tickets for hooligans. The available nutrients are also absorbed by the microbiome, so that the few survivors among the invaders no longer have any food available. To be on the safe side, our bacteria produce additional substances that render these pathogens harmless. All this together is a very effective combination of: Buying all the tickets, drinking all the beer, and if in doubt, pulling out a bottle of tear gas.

Diversity and Dysbiosis in the Realm of Microbes

Diversity is not only a dictum in companies that are looking for a wider range of employees. It is also the main criterion of a healthy and stable microbiome. It is not quantity alone, but above all the composition of as many different species as possible that makes our microbiome flexible and robust. If a multicultural approach to society makes sense anywhere, it is in our intestines. The more different species of bacteria it contains, the better they can complement each other and are therefore capable of completely different performances than a lonely and very heterogeneous group alone.

We inhabitants of the modern Western world, however, have a huge problem: the diversity of our microbiome has apparently declined sharply over the last few decades. The microbiota of primitive peoples or people in developing countries, on the other hand, looks quite different. Here, rich and poor are clearly interchanged - at least in this respect there is indeed some justice in the world. Of course, these people have quite different problems, which we certainly do not want to have ourselves, but in terms of the "diversity of the microbiome" they are currently far superior to us. If we lived with a small tribe in the rainforest or in Burkina Faso, we wouldn't have a shiny Audi or BMW in our garage, but we probably wouldn't have to worry about allergies, obesity, tooth decay, diabetes or heart disease. This seems strange to us, because we are actually convinced that we live a much healthier life than people in the second or third world. We never go hungry, and the hygienic conditions are not comparable to those in developing countries. So how did we manage to saddle ourselves with an armada of civilization diseases and a weakened microbiome?

In summary, our western lifestyle can be identified as the main culprit. Low-fiber food, the far too frequent use of antibiotics and an almost sterile life, beginning with birth by Caesarean section, have increasingly weakened our microbiome over the last century. The life's work of eminent scientists such as Alexander Fleming and Robert Koch was able to spare people terrible suffering and fatal diseases, but at the same time it led to the disappearance of the microbiome.

Diversity and microbial poverty are also hereditary. The mother's microbiome is transferred to her newborn at birth. This also explains the fatal downward spiral. We decimate our own microbiome and pass it on directly to our offspring, who in turn decimate it and pass it on to their own children. Many of these children are also given their first antibiotics before the age of three, at the exact time when the microbiome and immune system are formed.

The term "intestinal dysbiosis" has become established for a strongly reduced or disturbed microbiome. However, the definition is rather difficult, because it is not yet clear how a perfect microbiome should look like and when exactly a dysbiosis is present. The causes are also difficult to determine. The general decline of bacteria diversity in the western world and its presumed triggers are well known. Apart from this, microbiome research at the current state of the art is not yet able to say one hundred percent under which circumstances an unstable state develops in individual cases or how it can be prevented in a targeted manner. Humans are not machines - one person is a chain smoker and will live to be a hundred years old, while the other always pays attention to a healthy lifestyle and yet one terrible day is diagnosed with cancer.

A possible trigger of dysbiosis is several successive intestinal diseases, especially in connection with antibiotic treatments as "remedies". For example, antibiotic-associated colitis occurs when the bacterial diversity has been decimated by broad-spectrum antibiotics and the free spaces in the intestine are occupied by Clostridium Difficile, a pathogen.

Other factors that have been proven to influence our microbe community are stress and psychological strain. We are also poorer than people in developing countries in this respect, because we have to perform more and more from year to year and function perfectly around the clock. The industrialized countries' motor is a huge horde of diligent hamsters, pedaling at full throttle until the heart attack redeems them. We still go to work even when we have a bad cold, so as not to show any weakness, and only the burnout or heart attack forces us to shift down a gear - whereupon, in case of doubt, we are simply replaced by the next person who is still functioning well. But that's not all, we usually return the money we earn to the industry immediately. For example, when we once again reach for the ready-made product due to lack of time, instead of cooking fresh and eating real food. These industrially manufactured products are a nightmare for our microbiome. They contain plenty of microbe-damaging substances such as emulsifiers and sweeteners, but hardly any fiber. Thus they also contribute to the creeping destruction of our microbe friends.

The consequences of reduced diversity and dysbiosis are devastating. More and more widespread diseases have been associated with both since the discovery of the microbiome. The spectrum ranges from general metabolic disorders to severe mental illnesses and autoimmune diseases, including chronic inflammatory bowel diseases. Autoimmune diseases very often affect children. Along with cardiovascular diseases and cancer, they are one of the biggest problems of our time and severely restrict the quality of life of these unfortunate patients. The finely tuned mechanisms of the formation and development of immune cells seem to no longer function in more and more people. Parkinson's, Alzheimer's and depression also go hand in hand with a greatly reduced microbiome, although the connection is not immediately obvious. The open question is merely one of cause and effect - which came first, the decimated microbial community or the disease?

Bacteria-Human-Networking

Our intestinal bacteria are real superheroes: They exchange genes, produce messenger sub-stances and vitamins and probably even influence human emotions. Conversely, the mental well-being of humans also has an effect on their bacteria. Especially the omnipresent stress in our western world is extremely harmful not only for humans but also for their microbe friends.

Gut Feeling

Although there are still many unknowns, some theses are already relatively well proven. The bacteria in our intestines not only communicate diligently with each other, but also send messenger substances directly to our brain - and all this without WhatsApp. It is therefore more than likely that they can influence our emotions and perhaps even our actions in a very direct way, which is somewhat frightening. After all, we firmly believe that as humans we have a kind of free will. Even though this usually evaporates quite quickly when we pass the chocolate shelf. But our bacteria can do much more, just like real superheroes. They are actually capable of swapping their genes with each other. And not by mating and passing them on to their offspring, but more like " Do you need some wood? I'd have some wool for you in exchange!" (for all friends of the board game "The Settlers of Catan").

The three parties brain, intestine and microbiome are quite gossippy and constantly exchange information with each other. If this networking does not function properly, it has a detrimental effect on our entire psyche and the physical health associated with it. We all know and use phrases like "decide by gut feeling" or "I don't have a good feeling in my gut" without thinking about it further. What was subconsciously clear to us since long, can now actually be proven within the framework of microbiome research: The dream couple microbiome and intestine have a huge influence on our thinking and our emotions. That is why the microbiome-Anti-Diet is not limited to our eating habits, but also includes the factor of stress reduction.

Chat between Intestine and Brain

The brain is the control center for our thoughts and actions and enables emotions and our cognitive awareness. It controls the entire body and its functions with the help of commands that are transmitted through a complex system of billions of nerve cells. Accordingly, we are rightly particularly proud of its outstanding achievements. Today, the function of the brain can be observed quite vividly with the help of tomography. Not only humans are transparent nowadays, but also their brains can only hide few secrets from the public. For example, doctors can tell from the activity of individual brain areas whether their patient is happy or afraid.

However, the brain does not perform all these tasks alone, but communicates with the intestine in various ways. The vagus nerve is the direct connection between both organs and enables the transport of neurotransmitters and other messenger substances. At the same time, the intestine and brain communicate "wireless" via hormones and inflammatory molecules. In the past, it was assumed that this communication was rather one-way - brain to intestine. Still, it is now known that a huge amount of information is also sent from the intestine to the brain.

For a long time, the intestine was underestimated as an organ with simple mechanical functions. This has changed rapidly in recent years. The intestine is actually a kind of little brother to the brain. It has its own nervous system with about the same amount of nerve cells as the spinal cord, the enteric nervous system. The intestine performs all functions around digestion completely autonomously. Normally, the brain regulates it only slightly, sending about ten percent of its signals to the intestine. However, the intestine is very talkative and constantly lets the brain know what it is doing and how it is doing. This is why ninety percent of the information flows from the intestine to the brain. Our brain takes this information and processes it without us ever being aware of it - except in very special situations.

For example, the intestine sends signals such as "nausea" to the brain. For its part, the brain uses a clever method to process so much information. It memorizes recurring situations and is therefore able to react to them more quickly. A pirate copy of this design is used in computer science, where it is called "artificial neural network (KNN)". One can imagine the whole thing in the same way as trails in a meadow. The more often you use the same path, the easier it is to find it again, and the faster you get ahead. This memorization explains why, after a long night whose unpleasant end is closely linked to the consumption of large quantities of alcohol, we shudder at the mere sight or smell of alcohol for a long time and prefer to avoid it. This example from everyday life shows quite clearly how much communication from the intestines can actually influence our actions.

But the principle does not only apply to bad experiences. Probably a large part of our moments of well-being also comes from the gut. Whether we feel good or not depends on an enormous amount of information that is sent through the body every second of our lives. This information is spread in the form of signal substances, such as hormones. Such a hormone is like a small memo, it is for example produced by the thyroid gland and sent out with its message. The message can only arrive where there is a suitable receptor, that is the docking point. This can be right next door, as if school children were exchanging small pieces of paper with messages. Or even very far away, then the message must float in the bloodstream until it reaches the landing strip.

But the well-known hormone-producing organs are not the only ones that twitter diligently here. In fact, the largest accumulation of hormone-producing cells is found in the intestine. The vast amount of these endocrine cells (cells that release hormones into the bloodstream) is greater than all other endocrine organs combined [3]. The intestine is therefore able to send messages to the brain or to the rest of the body. At the same time, the intestine is the storage location for over 90 percent of the feel-good hormone serotonin. Intestinal bacteria such as Bifidobacterium infantis produce tryptophan and contribute this basic component to the production of serotonin. In the brain the hormone controls human behavior and emotions, in the intestine it stimulates the muscles. Surprisingly, taste and smell sensors are also located in the intestine, mainly directly on the endocrine cells [4]. So maybe we enjoy our food not only through the tongue but also through our intestines. So it is no longer an empty phrase when we speak of gut feeling. Nowadays it is scientifically proven that the intestines have an influence on our emotions - and vice versa.

Bowel Diseases and Stress

Stress is one of the worst risk factors of our time, and at the same time one that we can hardly escape. Although the most tedious jobs of the past have long since been automated or can be done in a fraction of the time with the help of machines, we spend a large part of our lives on the job. In a job that allows us to live a comfortable life, but really fulfills just a few happy people only.

The time of division of labor within the family is also over. With buzzwords such as emancipation and self-fulfillment, millions of women have been led to seek their happiness in working life and to expose themselves to the double burden of work and family. Whether we really want this deep down or whether we have just been manipulated to fuel both the economy and consumption, we will probably never know. Women in the western world have gained more independence and prestige with this change, but both partners pay for it with a chronically high level of stress.

If the job brings more stress than happiness, we want to enjoy life in our free time even more. To this end, we pack as much fun and activities as possible into the far too short hours after work and the measly weekend that we have earned with five days of work. We always have something on the agenda, are fully occupied and have no time for ourselves or to simply go for a long walk without looking at the clock. There's always something to buy that we absolutely must have, or something to do that you just must have done - of course not without days of research to really choose the best alternative. This is perfect for the economy, but very bad for us - and for our microbes.

It is possible that the course for our susceptibility to stress is set very early in life. Professor Emeran Mayer is investigating the effect of early childhood experiences on the dialogue between the intestines and the brain [5]. The general susceptibility to mental disorders is given to us from the time of conception until the age of eighteen. Anyone who had a happy childhood without trauma is very likely to be a relatively happy person later in life. This has been proven both in experiments with rats and in studies with human test persons. Test subjects who had traumatic experiences before the age of eighteen, such as verbal or physical abuse, a divorce of parents or the loss of a caregiver, had one thing in common, and that was a visible change in the salience network. This network is a part of the brain and determines how strongly we evaluate possible risks and dangers of a decision or the significance of an emotion. Due to their altered brain structure, the subjects were more risk-averse and anxious as adults, in other words more pessimistic overall than people who had a happy childhood.

Nature may have set this up so that creatures that are repeatedly exposed to life-threatening situations can cope particularly well with them. Our problem begins with the chronic stress of modernity, which our body interprets as "constant danger", although we are not actually exposed to any physical danger.

Now we pan the camera, away from the brain and towards the intestines, and then we move to the wide angle setting and look at both.

Under normal circumstances, the intestines work comfortably and autonomously, and the brain leaves them largely alone. But in emergency situations the big brother pushes the little brother aside and takes control. For example, the brain orders the stomach and intestines to empty more quickly, even in both directions at the same time, if the situation requires it. Anxiety and stress are such emergency situations, even though they are rarely life-threatening. We usually associate stress with too much workload or unpleasant situations, but inflammation or injury, pain, poor sleep and even menstruation are also stressors that can cause accelerated digestion.

This is perfectly fine as long as these emergency situations are limited to a few moments or short phases in our lives. But when we are chronically stressed, this does not only become a problem for our cardiovascular system. If our boss comes by every now and then to give us a new assignment or to ask what we are doing, that is not an issue. But if the boss stands behind us all day, gives us new orders every minute and constantly monitors us, we are no longer able to do our job properly. Probably it is similar to the intestine when its owner is under constant stress.

A large number of people nowadays suffer from intestinal problems. If it is not a disease with measurable or visible symptoms, such as inflammation of the bowel, both doctor and patient are usually at a loss. The diagnosis may then be "irritable bowel syndrome". In irritable bowel syndrome (IBS), a completely normal digestive process causes embarrassing and usually painful flatulence or cramps. The intestines of IBS patients therefore react completely inappropriately sensitively to ordinary stimuli. The brain behaves in a similar way in people with a correspondingly high level of stress. Mental illnesses and traumas produce a hypersensitive reaction to stress situations that other people put away quite easily.

This is precisely a very interesting insight. A very similar effect, namely the hypersensitive reaction to normal stimuli, can thus be detected simultaneously on both sides of the intestinal-brain axis. Psychological disorders such as overanxiety or depression are often associated with irritable bowel syndrome (IBS) in patients. The strong connection between brain and intestine via the vagus nerve and signal substances only partially explains this connection. However, there is a third component that creates a very special connection between the intestine and the brain.

Brain, Intestine and Microbiome - Ménage à Trois

Recent research is not limited to disorders of the intestinal-brain axis. Instead, it also involves the microbiome. The microbiome fills the gap between both types of problems, psychological disorders and intestinal diseases. Science is now working fervently to better understand the connections. The transplantation of stool is one of the methods used. It most clearly shows the direct effect of the microbiome and its metabolites. Not only the figure or health, but also the **nature** of mice (I cannot use enough exclamation marks at this point) can be transferred by stool transplantation to mice without their own microbiome (gnotobiotic animals). The microbiome of frightened mice turns gnotobiotic animals into frightened mice as well.

The stress hormone norepinephrine is another good example of such connections between the brain, intestine and microbiome. It not only raises blood pressure, but also reaches the intestines, where it can communicate directly with our bacteria friends. While our good bacteria unfortunately have their problems with norepinephrine, the harmful bacteria obviously get along well with this hormone. Their growth is stimulated, and with this newly gained superiority they can cause severe intestinal inflammation [6]. In the experiment with the gnotobiotic animals, the microbiome influences emotions, whereas in this example emotions have an effect on the microbiome.

Research into these interactions is more than interesting, which is why studies also aim to identify cause and effect, as does the study described above on the consequences of an unhappy childhood. In this study, despite trauma in childhood, not all patients had bowel problems, but only about half of them. An unhappy childhood does not necessarily lead to irritable bowel syndrome, but it is a risk factor.

However, stress has an additional negative influence on the microbiome. Stress and danger ensure that the intestine wants to get rid of its contents as quickly as possible. Diarrhea and a higher secretion of digestive juices are the result. Diarrhea is as catastrophic for our intestinal bacteria as a tsunami. The environment of our microbiome changes abruptly. This tsunami has a particularly harmful effect on the lactobacilli that are useful for us. The friendly squatters are washed away and make room for pathogens, which are also stimulated to greater aggressiveness by stress hormones [5]. Inflammatory intestinal diseases can be the result.

The altered microbiome now talks to the brain again and may be responsible for the occurrence of mental disorders. And so the circle is complete. Stress makes the intestine more sensitive to stimuli, the intestine then damages the microbiome, and the microbiome passes its distress on to the brain, triggering depression or other disorders.

In experiments with rats and mice, their susceptibility to stress and anxiety could be reduced by the intake of probiotics. There are also some smaller studies with people who have demonstrated a positive effect of probiotics from plain yogurt on the psyche. However, larger studies are still missing. If they ever do exist (and they certainly will), these studies will probably not be aimed at recommending a microbiome-friendly diet, but rather at the extremely lucrative sale of probiotics from online shops. But we don't have to wait for these studies and the products that come out of them. Because one thing can be said with certainty about microbe-friendly nutrition, and it is quite pragmatic: Whether or not its effect has been proven in studies, it has been tested over several million years and can in no way do any harm. Quite in contrast to the industrial food that is so widespread today.

Depression from the Intestine

The German Federal Ministry of Health writes on the subject of depression:

"Depressive disorders are among the most common and, in terms of their severity, most underestimated diseases. It is estimated that around 350 million people worldwide now suffer from depression. According to the World Health Organization, depression or affective disorders will be the second most common disease worldwide by 2020. [7]

Happiness researchers mainly blame our genes for whether or not we are naturally happy and optimistic. The inherited genes should have a share of at least 50 percent in our personal level of happiness. So you could say that pessimistic parents automatically produce other little pessimists with similar behavior and characteristics. The rest is determined by life circumstances and personal attitude. How do the genes manage to make us happy or unhappy? Genes don't actually "do" anything, they are just the equivalent of the IKEA assembly instructions. The gene tells our body what it should do. Some of these genes control the uptake of serotonin and thus the amount of the available serotonin in our blood. Serotonin deficiency is associated with depression. For example, the Danes seem to be a particularly happy people and have been shown to have genes that promote high serotonin levels [8]. If this serotonin level is very low, genetically or otherwise, and depression makes life difficult, doctors and pharmacists can help. One of the most effective mood-lifting chemicals are serotonin reuptake inhibitors. These drugs increase the amount of serotonin in the bloodstream.

In summary, there are two factors that have an effect on depression, the serotonin storage capacity, or availability in the blood, and the building blocks of our genes. In this context, let us go back to our microbiota. Serotonin and genes are responsible for our happiness. Since over 90 percent of serotonin is stored in the intestine, it is more than likely that the intestine and our microbiome play a major role when it comes to depression - and vice versa. Also, most of the genes in our body do not come from ourselves, but from the microbiome. Different people do not differ so much in their own genes, but their microbiomes do. Suspicion springs to mind, that our microbes play a far greater role in emotions, feelings of happiness, depression or psychological disorders than we had previously thought. Microbe-friendly nutrition has the potential to enhance our quality of life by strengthening our immune system, but also by providing a more positive bundle of emotions.

Fast Healing -
Made Easy?

The body can heal itself very well if we support it a little bit. The microbiome is an important component of this support, which we are kind enough provided free of charge. However, there is also this one precious ingredient that we actually never have at home: time...

Self-Help by Shopping

The 30-day Anti-Diet gives you an idea of what a microbe-friendly nutrition that is also suitable for everyday use could look like. However, this single month is of course not enough to eliminate all the health problems that have accumulated in recent years forever. Self-healing with the microbiome is a long and ongoing process. A little self-discipline, commitment and perseverance are indeed necessary to say goodbye to some old habits and try something new. Not to mention more exercise and active stress reduction. Of course, the whole thing has to be kept up in the long run. It goes forward in small steps, but sometimes also a step back again, for example when the stress level is higher.

That's what we all hate to hear. For most people, it's not enough actionism and it takes too long. We would like to swallow one capsule and see the result the next day, reliable like an Amazon prime order. This is where the advertising machinery of the "health industry" comes in, and very successfully - for the industry, not for us.

Sick people are of course looking for remedies to cure themselves and are willing to spend large sums of money and a lot of time on it and even try out very experimental "insider tips". In the field of intestinal diseases, it is downright frustrating how little help the patient receives from the doctor.

Conventional medicine does a great job and we should be glad every day that it exists. However, it performs its best services more in the field of mechanics. Destroyed bones can be repaired miraculously and with the help of the regenerative power of our body. Even tumors can be removed better and better. If the heart beats too fast, it can be slowed down, if it beats irregularly, the pacemaker helps. We cannot do without all this.

However, especially in the area of intestinal diseases, which are becoming more and more widespread, no major advances in medicine have yet been seen from the patients' perspective. Either the patient is more or less subtly labelled as a hypochondriac, or the treatment is limited to a temporary relief of the symptoms before they reappear with full force and sometimes even more severely.

Therefore, the widespread skepticism towards conventional medicine in this particular field is not surprising. The afflicted are looking for alternatives, even if it is only the alternative practitioner who at least listens to them, instead of releasing them from the treatment room after five minutes with a prescription and a "If it doesn't get better, come back again". However, some of the methods advertised as alternative and natural medicine are sometimes adventurous, and their usefulness is questionable.

Lucrative Health Industry

In every area of our lives there are critics who cannot and will not accept the circumstances and the restrictions on our freedom and health. In the area of health these critics often find themselves as opponents of orthodox medicine and buyers of mysterious roots, berries or powders. These miracle cures should make us healthy, slim and beautiful within a few weeks.

A huge industry has built up around this myth. Tremendous amounts of money are made with the hope and suffering of many people. The only one who is helped by this is the respective seller of these miracle cures, just like the travelling quack in the Wild West back then. Nowadays, sales are handled more elegantly, via online platforms and unknown manufacturers. This approach minimizes the risk of leaving the city tarred and feathered. Doctors and consumer protection agencies are at a loss in the fight against this industry. No matter how emphatically they point out that taking dietary supplements is unnecessary, this industry is booming.

The advertising behind these dubious products is financed with a lot of money and works with numerous psychological tricks. Therefore, no one need be embarrassed if they have already bought such magic beans themselves. I myself was no different from my fellow sufferers in search of help. I googled the relevant sites (for example the German online portal "Center of Health"), found a lot of interesting information that sounds very plausible, and ... shopped like crazy.

Grapefruit extract, wheatgrass powder, acerola powder and apple pectin ended up in my shopping cart, I even can't remember everything. Thank God humans repress many things in the course of their lives. We want to be slim and healthy, if possible without eating less or eating healthier food or getting more exercise, and if there is even the slightest chance that a capsule eaten daily will do the trick, then we buy it. Or even several, just in case...

But unfortunately after some time we have to realize we were tricked. None of these mysterious remedies actually help, and if they do, then at most through the placebo effect, i.e. our firm belief in an impact. Because in contrast to these various remedies, our body is a real miracle. If it is not too weakened and if it is not hindered, our body heals itself. From a scientific point of view, this is the only plausible explanation for the fact that some people report an improvement of their symptoms after taking a "medicine" without any provable effect. Probably during this time the body healed itself, supported by a firm faith which is known to move mountains. A popular argument is the healing of animals after taking the "miracle weapon". Animals also possess self-healing powers, and even an animal will certainly notice if its human being cares a little more about the animal and treats it with a little more love. So why should self-healing and additional care not have any influence on animals?

Mysterious Miracle Remedies

We are in one of the relevant online shops on the subject of health. The webpage title promises us exactly what we are longing for: "Everything the body needs - just one click away!" [9]. The product groups are divided into the topics that move us most. Losing weight - who wouldn't want to lose weight in a world that offers so much abundance and so little compulsion to move, but at the same time propagates an unattainable ideal of beauty? Detox, the buzzword par excellence. Somehow we feel constantly poisoned, especially when we surf such websites, and we absolutely must do something about it. Acid-base balance - for the followers of the acidosis theory. Digestion, one of the most critical topics of modern times, because more and more people have quite some problems with it. Vitamins, minerals and vitality in general. Which vitamin group should I choose? B, C, D, E, K, or rather a whole vitamin complex? For losing weight there is a colorful bouquet of appetite suppressants, fat burners and food-like substances, like Michael Pollan would express it [10], for example, sugar substitute and noodles without carbohydrates.

With cures, alkaline foods, alkaline teas, alkaline body care and alkaline water we should be able to achieve the perfectly balanced acid-base body - hey guys, am I a chemistry set, or what? According to advertisements, digestion can be improved quite easily with the help of dietary fibers, prebiotics and probiotics (of course, each as separate products, not in the form of simple healthy food) and creepy methods of intestinal cleansing. Descriptions of detox and purification cures point out that without them our body is gradually poisoned and we are hopelessly lost. With a glance at the list of minerals on offer, it is perfectly clear to us that we certainly have far too little of them, and that every day. As if all this wasn't enough, we should also be concerned about our eye health, oxidizing cells, healthy sleep, stomach, kidneys, immune system and mood. The thing with the good mood and healthy sleep will be over at the latest when we look at this mountain of "must have products" and roughly calculate the monthly costs of this seemingly perfect healthy life in capsule and powder form. Apart from the fact that we would probably already have covered our daily calorie requirements after taking all these products. Let's pick out a few examples.

Wheatgrass juice powder, just under forty euros for a can of 200 grams. Quote: "Cereal grasses and the juice powder made from these grasses should no longer be missing in any health-conscious household [11]. Of course we are health-conscious, otherwise we would not be here. So off to the shopping cart with the miracle cure from the USA - the country that is known worldwide for its insanely healthy inhabitants. Just to let you know, wheatgrass juice tastes like whisked duck poop. It was part of my personal miracle cure phase a few years ago, so I can tell you about it. After buying the green powder I was a little poorer. Surprisingly, I didn't become slimmer, more beautiful or healthier by choking it down.

"Simsalabim Cassis" provides for a "clever slimming experience". Not a nasty torture, but a weight loss experience! Since an experience itself can't be clever at all, it naturally implies that the buyer of the product is particularly clever. Quite contrary to the hopeless dumb-asses who want to lose weight with the help of abstinence and more exercise, we do this quite simply with a vegan diet shake for just under 25 euros per can of 500 gram. Simsalabim, hocuspocus, and we are slim and can still sit on our couch and eat burgers with fries. Of course, this miracle cure is also "perfectly suited for year-round weight management" - so it's best to buy several packs at once!

The better alternative: Be really clever and eat the "high-quality proteins from rice and peas" simply in the form of much cheaper rice and peas...

Sango Sea Coral with Zinc & Silicon, 120 capsules for 25 bucks - the daily dose is four capsules. According to advertising, the nutrients contained in the coral contribute "among other things" to the normal acid-base balance, support healthy hair, skin and nails and the psychological function. Whatever a "normal acid-base balance" is. But since this is not really clear, we simply have to assume that our body is somehow in a state of imbalance, comparable to the national budget of most countries in the world.

We read all these cleverly devised descriptions and then believe that if we don't buy all the hocuspocus stuff, we are practically no longer viable. This is not because we are particularly stupid, but because of sophisticated advertising methods that take advantage of our human weaknesses and ways of thinking. For example, the widespread fear of accumulating toxins and waste products in the body, especially in the intestines.

Our Intestine in Guantanamo

Whether recommended by alternative practitioners or self-prescribed, intestinal cleansing is a trend, and not just since yesterday. Even in ancient times, people in many different cultures around the world suspected that horrible things were accumulating in their intestines that had negative effects on health and therefore definitely had to be removed. The ancient Egyptians were as obsessed with this idea as the Sumerians, Babylonians, Assyrians, Indians, Chinese, Koreans and Greeks. For example, Hippocrates himself was convinced of the positive effects of enemas [12]. Nowadays we smile at many other beliefs of that time. For example, today we are fully aware that the world is not a disc. But the riddle of the poisoned intestine has remained with us until today. Fired by the health industry, which is making a killing with this misconception. Let's go back to our sample shop and see what is offered there for the removal of residues in the intestines and what absurd claims are made there.

Cat Litter and Overpriced Sugar

Bentonite, a central component of intestinal cleansing, "wanders through the intestine like a kind of "garbage chute" and is supposed to bind heavy metals, pesticides and other "unwanted pollutants" (By the way, it is also practical for use in garden ponds). It goes without saying that it is an integral part of life for health-conscious people, must not be missing in any medicine chest and of course is suitable for almost everyone - anything else would be detrimental to the seller's business. This miracle weapon comes from the USA and is called so because it was allegedly found near Fort Benton [13]. We also know bentonite from another application in which the use of bentonite is actually useful: In the litter box. So it's best to leave the stuff there instead of eating it.

Yacon root powder, a "wonderful and above all delicious alternative to conventional granulated sugar" - at a price of incredible 99.30 euros per kilogram. For comparison: One kilogram of normal household sugar of the German noble brand Südzucker costs 1.36 euro. A certain skepticism as to whether the cake with yacon root powder actually tastes as good as the cake with normal sugar is appropriate. However, according to the advertisement, the powder, unlike household sugar, is prebiotic, with 9.6 grams of dietary fiber per 100 grams of powder, and also contains 130 mg potassium, 2.9 mg iron and 150 mg phosphorus. And already the first doubts arise whether we should not try it after all, and whether it wouldn't be worth the money.

Just relax. There is a very simple, cheaper and much healthier alternative: Replace 100 grams of the flour in the recipe with wholemeal flour. 100 grams of wholemeal wheat flour contain: 10 grams of fiber, at least 17 different vitamins, 13 minerals and trace elements, of which 381 mg potassium, 3.3 mg iron and 341 mg phosphorus) plus amino acids [14]. There is no question that sugar is not particularly healthy, so let's simply use ten or twenty percent less sugar. This works quite well for most cakes, even if the consistency may suffer a little bit. A normal fruitcake base then still contains 80 grams of sugar. Normally, however, you don't eat the cake all by yourself, but share this amount of sugar with 11 other people. Of course, this also applies to the dietary fibers and minerals, but I would still rather not recommend eating the whole cake alone. Every day there are numerous other ways to cover the need for fiber and to make the intestinal bacteria happy.

Coffee - In a Whole New Way!

Swallowing fiber and cat litter in capsule form is generally something for sissies. Of course, the truly health-conscious person does not stop halfway, but does everything at once, with highly efficient intestinal cleansing. Intestinal cleansing in general is practically advertised as indispensable on our sales platform, with sentences like these:

"To understand what a bowel cleansing is all about, one may compare this traditional method with a big cleaning of the largest and most important digestive organ of the human body. During intestinal cleansing, food residues, slag and other harmful substances are removed from the intestine and the intestinal flora is brought back into balance. [...] By cleaning the intestines, digestive problems can be remedied, the immune system strengthened and thus the overall well-being optimized.

The reader involuntarily thinks "Oh my God, I have to go and clean my bowels immediately before something bad happens". The advertisement for intestinal cleansing is followed by a longer explanation why the intestine is so important. The explanation is of course correct, the intestine is definitely important. However, the claim that there are food residues and waste products in the intestine is nothing but humbug. However, since the corresponding "cures" are sold as food supplements, they are not subject to any drug approval. In advertising, just about anything can be claimed, including the claim that the day after taking the magic pills, a unicorn will be at your doorstep. Safety, quality and effectiveness are tested by the manufacturer alone. Any suspicion is unreservedly appropriate.

An even worse idea is probably the colonic hydrotherapy, also called colonic irrigation. Now at the latest everyone should know what is meant. No matter how medically, clinically or neutrally you express it and talk about "gentle cleansing and stimulation", the fact is: You voluntarily pump liquids into your butt that really don't belong there, like coffee or green tea. The procedure is of course once again "no longer an insider tip in health-conscious circles". We are apparently the only ones who have obviously not yet received this important information. That's why we still live with our imaginary, but still pretty disgusting intestinal deposits (which, by the way, is called "slags" in Germany).

Although the intestine definitely contains no obscure residues or deposits, it is home to countless microorganisms that live with us - for better or worse. Of course, not all the microbes that are in our intestines are our friends. That is why it is important to support the good bacteria and help them to become numerous and strong enough to give the harmful ones a good kick in the ass. However, the colonic irrigation flushes away everything, good and bad bacteria, and damages our microbiome.

Even long fasting is not entirely uncritical. A short fasting cure may sometimes be quite appropriate and beneficial, but longer fasting means malnutrition for our intestinal bacteria. The starving microbes have only one alternative as a substitute food - the intestinal mucosa.

An excessive starvation diet is therefore probably not the best thing for our healthy intestines, not to mention this deluge story.

Integrated Cleaning Function - Free and Effective

On the one hand, this fear of toxins in the intestines is understandable. The intestine is indeed the cause of many problems, and from the point of view of the sufferer it is not possible to understand what exactly the cause is. We can't just take a quick look inside the intestine. It sometimes gargles frighteningly, pinches and cramps, inflates painfully or very hesitantly reveals its contents - or the opposite. Even modern medicine is still largely in the dark when it comes to intestinal diseases - in the truest sense of the word. However, not as far as the presence of digestive waste (in Germany, it is called "slags") or other deposits in the intestine is concerned. So writes Dr. Werner Bartens:

"No one can answer what exactly is meant by intestinal cleansing. No researcher has so far succeeded in detecting waste products (slags) in the body or in the laboratory. [...] Even the talk of acidosis is nonsense. Our cells and organs work at a fairly constant pH. There is no need

to restore the basis balance. The only thing that can throw you off balance is the rip-off." [15]

When the gastrologist looks at the intestine during the dreaded colonoscopy, he normally sees a beautiful pinkish structure. Clean as a whistle and without ominous intestinal deposits and dirt globules that would have been deposited somewhere. There are, of course, diseases where the sight is not so pleasant. Inflammatory bowel diseases, carcinomas, polyps and diverticula make the beautiful pink landscape a living nightmare. But these are all symptoms that the gastrologist discovers during his examination and can treat accordingly.

A perhaps somewhat unscientific, but still relatively credible proof of the fairy tale of the cinders - for all those who don't have an endoscope at home: Let's just google " intestinal deposits" and switch on the image search. But be careful, this is not for the faint of heart!

There is actually nothing in the world for which there is no picture on Google, except for the intestinal deposits that are repeatedly cited. When we search, we find pictures of inflamed intestines or just disgusting pictures of garbage lying around somewhere. But if we were all constantly poisoned internally and plagued by deposits in the intestines, wouldn't we be swarming with pictures showing these deposits?

They do not exist, and for one simple reason. The stomach and intestines cleanse themselves. It happens with the help of a really cool function, the migrating motor complex. First the stomach and then the intestines contract with a lot of force and squeeze their contents towards the exit, like a toothpaste tube. Our body repeats this process diligently and reliably over and over again, every one and a half to three hours. When the stomach is empty, the growling sound that we all know and which is so embarrassing at the wrong moment is produced. Only when the motor complex no longer functions properly do we have to worry about cleaning our intestines. This does not just happen, however, but is connected with serious illnesses such as diabetes.

Fraud on the Buyer

Many people believe steadfastly in their personal favorite products or ways to health and react indignantly to any kind of skepticism. In principle, this is fine - not everything in the world has to be scientifically explainable and faith of any kind is usually characterized by the absence of evidence. To be fair, the lack of proof does not necessarily mean that something does not exist.

Not so long ago, people would have said that the presence of tiny creatures on our bodies was the fantasy of a lunatic. Before the microscope was invented, there was no way of proving the existence of bacteria, but bacteria did exist. We still do not know everything, and certainly many unknown remedies of all kinds will appear in the course of our further history. But some of them seem to be quite far-fetched. When someone tells me that

I have to dissolve a shot glass of beer in a jug of water to get a hundred times drunk as with undiluted beer, I am rather skeptical. But millions of homeopathy followers believe in this principle. Perhaps one day a scientific explanation for the effectiveness of homeopathic remedies will be found, and all those who until then had been ridiculed for their beliefs will perhaps be able to say: "I always knew it! Dear followers of homeopathy, if the effectiveness of homeopathic remedies can ever be scientifically proven, I hereby apologize prophylactically for my unjustified assertions.

Natural remedies are another category, although they are often lumped together with homeopathic remedies. Mankind knew how to help itself even before the emergence of large pharmaceutical companies, and the effectiveness of various natural remedies has been proven. It is not necessary to pull out the chemical mace immediately if you feel sick. It can't hurt to have natural remedies as the first wave of attack against common simple sicknesses and ailments in the home.

When it comes to the numerous miracle cures in online shops and pharmacies, however, a certain mistrust is appropriate. These are not necessarily natural remedies. While the benefits of natural active ingredients are quite verifiable, this is generally not the case with modern miracle drugs. Nevertheless, these products are not explicitly advertised with the statement "the effect is not verifiable", instead the sellers want to make us believe the opposite. In this case one can speak of deliberate fraud. Nicholas Nassim Taleb describes the situation very aptly: "We have managed to transfer religious belief into gullibility for whatever can masquerade as science." [16].

These various powders, capsules, liquids and tablets are summarized under the group "food supplements". In contrast to pharmaceuticals, they are not subject to any mandatory approvals [17]. Not only do most products have to be called placebo when viewed soberly, some of them even contain extremely harmful substances. The consumer is lied to with dubious stories about the discovery and origin of the products. However, these pseudo drugs are not brewed by the forest elves, but are partly sold by the same pharmaceutical companies that also produce orthodox medicine - or even worse, by completely unknown companies around the world. It is rather unlikely that an old, wise Indian on his deathbed quickly passed on his ancestors' ancient recipe for a healthy intestine to one of these pharmaceutical companies.

For the ultimate healing from faith in miracle cures and so called insider tips, reading the (German) magazine "Gute Pillen - Schlechte Pillen" (*Good Pills - Bad Pills*) is very helpful [18]. The editorial team is made up of doctors, pharmacists, health scientists and other natural scientists. It works independently of the pharmaceutical industry and takes a critical look at the products that are advertised to us in our search for a better and healthier life. After reading ten or twenty issues at the latest, one thing becomes perfectly clear: there is no such thing as a miracle remedy for this and that. We are only being deceived, and on a massive scale.

A Stronger Microbiome in 30 Days - Is that Possible?

The microbiome of a hunter-gatherer tens of thousands of years ago would laugh out loud at our small, weak microbiome. The diversity of our intestinal bacteria is severely decimated, and so far no means of adding new species permanently are known. This makes it all the more important to provide optimal support for the remaining microbiome. Because our microbe friends are extraordinarily adaptable.

Grandma Hedwig's Hut

First the bad news: Those who live in the western world have inherited a western microbiome along with western culture. Unfortunately, not every inheritance gives cause for rejoicing, some just inherit the decayed little hut with outhouse from granny Hedwig. It is a similar story with our microbiome in a world that is characterized by disinfection and antibiotics, chronic stress, industrially produced food and births by caesarean section. During the first three years of life our intestinal bacteria develop into a closed society which does not accept new members for the rest of our lives, but in case of doubt can lose some, for example through the use of antibiotics. The microbiome of primitive peoples differs greatly from ours in its biodiversity, while the microbiomes of all western people are very similar. One would actually expect that a German vegan has completely different species of bacteria than a passionate Austrian meat eater, but surprisingly this is not the case. It looks like we have to live in our hut with an outhouse and can't even turn it into a villa with a pool by an extreme change of diet.

Because of the limited diversity, our microbiome is less stable and therefore more vulnerable to problems, just like any other ecosystem. Even if we eat plenty of fruit and vegetables, our intestinal bacteria can make less useful substances from them than the microbes of the Stone Age hunter. With the gradual change in human lifestyle, man has lost this source of health forever unless science can restore it in the future. However, we will hardly be able to wait that long.

But there is also good news. Although a dietary change unfortunately cannot restore the extinct species, it seems to have a very large influence on the microbiome in other ways. Nutrition changes the environment of our intestinal bacteria and they react to it.

Rapid Adaptation through Exponential Growth

Every adaptation in the microbiome happens at lightning speed. Bacteria have an interesting and very effective method of multiplying. They simply divide, without any partner search or an evening with wine and candlelight. The second bacterium is an exact copy of the first, with all its genes. Both bacteria regenerate after division and become the next generation. E. coli bacteria can divide about every 20 minutes and create 72 copies of themselves per day [19]. But that's not all it is. At this point, one thing comes into play that some of us still remember gloomily from mathematics lessons - the exponential function. The exponential function describes a growth process like that of our bacteria and forms a steep upward curve.

If only a single bacterium were to duplicate itself again and again while its offspring remained inactive, the result would look like this after 24 hours:

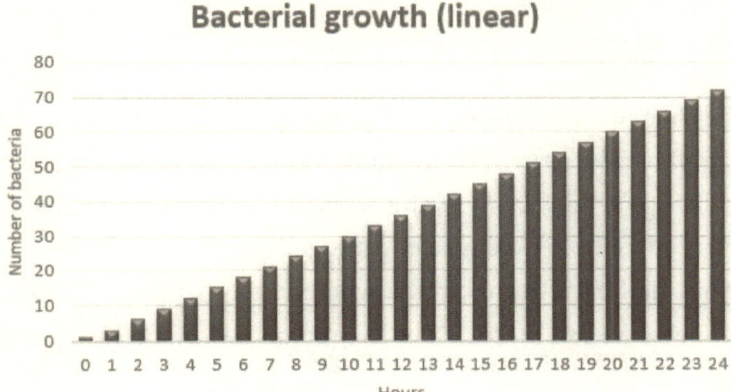

Notional doubling without "compound interest"

This fact alone would be quite impressive. A single bacterium can produce 72 bacteria in just one day! However, this does not yet take into account the fact that the newly formed bacteria not only hang around lazily, but also multiply diligently under reasonably favorable conditions. And this is where the exponential function comes in, the effect of which is so difficult for our minds to understand, although it is so important for us in real life.

The microbes in and on our bodies don't really care whether we can mathematically calculate their growth rates. But the exponential function also unfolds its enormous power in the case of interest rates and inflation, and here we really should take a closer look. As far as bacterial growth is concerned, the effect of exponential function is not only fascinating, but it also explains why the intestinal microbiome can actually adapt to changes in a very short time. Every 20 minutes, the respective number of bacteria doubles, and each new generation has the opportunity to adapt to the environment a little better.

The most vivid example of this principle comes from the story with the chessboard and the grain of rice - even the king could not imagine how many grains of rice were on the last square. If after only 6 hours we would get together not only the children of our first bacterium, but the whole family with all nieces and nephews and so on for a family photo, the whole thing would look like this:

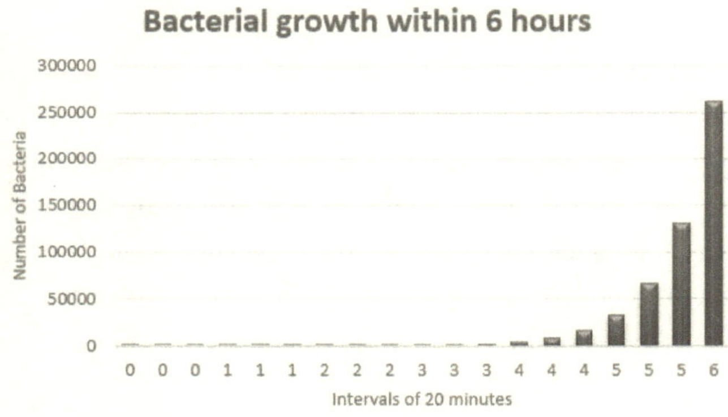

Doubling by division - three times per hour

262,144 microbes would cuddle up for the photo. But here we are still in the "uncritical" part of the exponential function, where it is still somewhat flat when you look at the whole picture.

After only 24 hours, the number of bacteria is so large that it can only be read by mathematicians: 4.72236648286965E+21, which is roughly a 4.7 with 21 zeros behind it. While Scrooge Duck might have called it multiplujillion, quadrillion is the mathematical name. We don't care, because to be honest, neither of them mean anything to us. At the latest in the billion range, the figures are no longer tangible for us. The following graphic shows the corresponding bacterial growth.

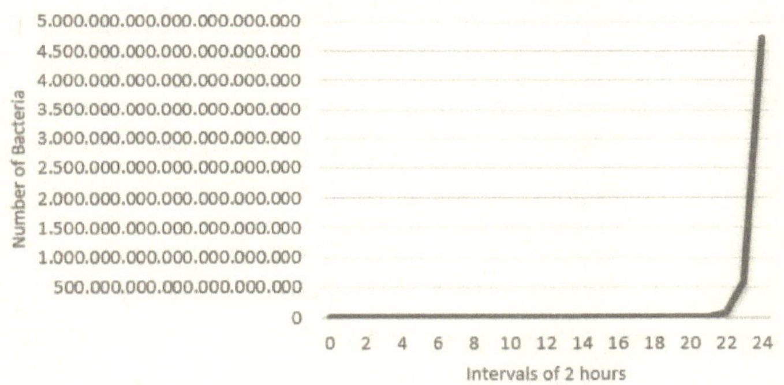

Doubling by division - three times per hour

The number of deceased is not included. The small creatures are quite resilient, but if they were to multiply at this rate in our intestines and survive for several days, we would explode quite quickly. So, life and death are apparently in balance. Regardless of whether we can still read these numbers or understand the exponential function, this incredible growth rate shows above all how quickly our bacteria can adapt to changes. Damn quickly...

Flexible in the Choice of Job

A bacteria community is very flexible. Whole groups of bacteria can take over tasks of missing groups as long as the missing groups are not key species. In case of doubt, our bacteria friends even exchange genes with other bacteria and take over their properties and abilities with the genes, like superheroes in a Marvel comic. Genes that a microbe already possesses can be activated or deactivated, as required. If the gene for heat resistance is not needed - get rid of it! It would only be unnecessary ballast. But in case the bacterium happens to be lying on the beach around lunchtime, it can activate the gene again. Nevertheless, new species will never be added, except for those that are created by gene exchange. But it doesn't seem to matter much what kind of bacteria we harbor, because, as already mentioned, they can perform their tasks very flexibly. The more different species, the better, but even a less diverse microbiome can still perform its tasks quite well to a certain extent.

A change in diet does not affect diversity, but the group size of different existing species may change. It is now known, for example, that obesity is associated with a higher number of Firmicutes species, while Bacteroides species are declining in number. When eating a high-fat diet, the liver produces more bile, which also migrates to the intestines. Bacteria that tolerate bile acid therefore feel particularly well, while other species are reduced [20]. Nutrition and overweight therefore have an influence on the composition of the intestinal bacteria. Conversely, however, the "overweight" microbiome also causes people to gain even more weight - a vicious circle. This influence of the microbiome has been proven several times with the help of laboratory mice, one of the first big sensations in microbiome research. If a slim mouse is given the microbiome of a fat mouse via a stool transplantation, the bikini body quickly becomes a burqa body. With exactly the same food intake, mice with a "chubby" microbiome gain weight, while their conspecifics with a slim microbiome remain slim.

Fortunately, we are not lab mice. We can usually choose for ourselves what we eat and which bacteria we support particularly well. Together with our intestinal bacteria, we can influence whether we become fat or thin.

Advantage through Metabolites. Meta... what?

A healthy bacterium will eat anything we put before it. However, for this to happen, the meal must arrive at the bacterium and not be processed in the digestive system beforehand. When a living being eats something, something comes out of the same living being, even if the living being is very small. Animal owners and parents of babies can certainly painfully confirm this. In the case of microorganisms, this "something" is not called poop, but metabolite. The good thing about these metabolites is that they can be useful to us. From carbohydrates, for example, our bacteria can produce short-chain fatty acids that care for our intestinal mucosa. However, the effect of the microbiome is not limited to the intestine. Up to 40 percent of the molecules in our blood are products of our intestinal microbiota [6]. In this way, the trillions of bacteria are able to send signals to the entire body, including the brain. It is very likely that our intestinal bacteria can control our emotions and perhaps even our behavior.

It is precisely at this point that a change in diet brings about the greatest change. Let's recap: The bacterial species in our intestines have been stable since the age of three, they are our legacy. We do not all have the same species, but microbiomes in industrial society generally have less diversity than those of primitive peoples. However, we can influence the respective proportion of species with our diet.

However, the biggest difference is in the excretion products of the microbes, the metabolites. Although it is the same species of bacteria in slightly different compositions that digest plant fibers in the vegan and proteins in the meat eater, their metabolites differ greatly. Dr. Emeran Mayer uses a wonderful comparison to illustrate this principle, an orchestra. A particular orchestra contains more or less the same types of musicians each time. One group each of violinists, plucked instruments, flutes, and so on. But this does not mean that these musicians always play the same song, otherwise the concert would be quite boring. The orchestra is fed with notes. The outcome is completely unique for each composition. Our microbiome works in exactly the same way If we feed it differently, the result will also change. Even with such a small change in our eating habits as the regular consumption of simple probiotic yogurt, a change in metabolites can be measured [6].

Changing Food Trends for the Microbe Community

Thanks to exponential growth and high flexibility, it is therefore possible to achieve a certain change in our inner microbe society and its metabolites within a short period of time. This was particularly important for our ancestors. If you have a grandmother or even great-grandmother, you should ask her what she had to eat in winter. Although her youth was only two or three generations ago, her diet has changed rapidly in that short time.

Suppose our grandmother lived in a country with a moderate climate and four seasons. At that time, no strawberries were flown in from the other side of the world in winter. There were no pineapples, no citrus fruits and all the other exotic fruits that have become a matter of course for us. Instead, the general diet was adapted to the seasons, and it was very local. In spring, freshly harvested salads from their own garden were on the menu. In late spring, our grannies ate strawberries and rhubarb and in summer juicy cherries and tomatoes. In autumn, a colorful bouquet of local fruit and root vegetables enriched the menu. During winter, our dear great-grandmother did not take the vegetables from the supermarket just because nothing grows in the garden. Instead, there were vegetables and fruit that could be stored, canned or fermented in the cool cellar. Like a very famous German classic with a strong smell, called "Sauerkraut".

One could assume that a drastic change in diet four times a year would be quite a strain on the body. After all, nowadays we are constantly being told that we should definitely eat a "balanced" and "regular" diet throughout the year. So how could humans survive for millions of years, even though until a few decades ago they were forced to go through long periods of hunger and otherwise ate completely different food groups depending on the season?

In order to optimally process this extremely variable food supply, the microbiota must adapt to the conditions, including in its composition. This is because not all bacteria use the same components of our food. Some bacteria are particularly good at metabolizing carbohydrates. Others manage to convert protein into vitamins.

Winds of Change

A change in the intestinal flora can be both positive and negative. If we normally eat a low-fat diet with lots of vegetables, but change to a very high-fat and low-fiber diet during holidays or over Christmas, the composition of the microbial community in our intestines will inevitably adapt during this time. But the same applies in the opposite case. The Microbiome-Anti-Diet should therefore definitely have an effect within a short period of time. The first physical change that becomes noticeable when switching to more dietary fiber is most likely a slightly higher gas production in the microbes' home. This may not necessarily be the desired effect at all, but it is nevertheless a sign that a change is taking place in a world invisible to us.

However, at this point, one suspicion naturally already suggests itself: It is not enough to follow the Microbiome-Anti-Diet for 30 days and then feast the rest of the year with impunity and unrestrained. But even these few days can help, for example, to compensate for a gourmet holiday or support the immune system after an illness. The 30-day approach is certainly also useful to support the immune system after a disease, especially after taking antibiotics, after a colonoscopy, after diarrhea or gastrointestinal tract diseases. All in all, however, they should only be a small inspiration for the rest of our lives. With its relaxed approach, the Microbiome Anti-Diet shows that we can simply eat a little healthier without tormenting ourselves daily or having to switch to dietary food forever.

All this can be done in a completely relaxed manner, with a lot of joy and love for real food. Forget the vegan raw vegetable platter and steamed market vegetables without fat and salt - there is a much more delicious way. There is no need to ban all existing supplies from the house or to leave the house with endless shopping lists just to support the microbiome.

Little Influencers

Not only our diet has an influence on the intestinal flora, but also the brain, which is in active communication with the nervous system of the intestine and our intestinal bacteria. That is why relaxation is a component of the Anti-Diet. In addition, taking probiotics - living bacteria - in capsule form could help, but it is not obligatory. There have been too few studies and evidence for this so far, so everyone has to decide for themselves whether they believe in the effects of probiotic capsules.

The main goal is to build up the intestinal flora. Achieving this goal, however, has other beneficial side effects, such as strengthening the immune system. 30 days is a very short time, so of course miracles are not to be expected. There may be only tiny differences, which you may not even notice directly. To say otherwise would be highly doubtful. But if you do something good for your microbiome more often afterwards, you will find out over time that these tiny changes do not stop there.

Your personal preferences will change over time. At some point you may find that fresh wholemeal bread actually tastes better than rolls made from white flour, and that the sight of a crispy leek suddenly gives you great ideas for dinner. The microbiome communicates with us. Perhaps a healthy microbiome shows its human being what is good for both if it is strong enough and if it is heard.

This book is intended as an introduction and small sample and hopefully makes you want more: More health, good mood and well-being for us and our intestinal bacteria. Healthy food must taste delicious and be fun instead of frustrating, otherwise the whole thing makes no sense.

Anti-Diet Part 1: Relax!

"Relaxation" is the first key word and the first big challenge. Away with endless shopping lists, the far too ambitious athletic program, a daily schedule with five meals, strict rules and all that stuff. A change in diet that causes more stress than we already have can't be healthy.

Microbe-Burnout

Some things are very easy for us once we have tried them, while others are among our weaknesses. The thing with relaxation is the hardest for me personally. Although I notice again and again how tense and stressed I walk through life, I rarely manage to allow myself the much-needed rest. I am certainly not alone with this problem. But there are good possibilities to get away from the hectic pace of everyday life, at least temporarily, and take life a little easier. Avoiding or reducing chronic stress is one of the most important points in supporting the microbiome, because stress is really bad for us and our bacteria friends.

Not everyone is equally susceptible to stress. While one person effortlessly completes all the tasks at hand, another person breaks out in a cold sweat at the very thought of the day ahead. Since science has been working on the microbiome, we know a few trillion other reasons why these differences exist.

Bowel diseases and increased susceptibility to stress are often related. We have known for a long time that chronic stress "makes someone's stomach turn". There are two relatively new findings from microbiome research. Intestinal diseases and increased susceptibility to stress are often related. We have known for a long time that chronic stress "makes someone's stomach turn over". There are two relatively new findings from microbiome research. First, mental strain causes the microbiome to change its composition, which explains why our digestive system suffers from stress. Secondly, our body releases certain hormones under stress, and microbiologists have been able to show that these hormones also reach the intestines, where they communicate directly with our bacteria. So our bacteria friends get lots of little text messages saying "Stress!", " Stress!", " Stress!", " Stress!"

Unfortunately it seems to be the case that of all things the bacteria that are harmful to us are attracted by this stress, like at a heavy metal concert, which attracts many peaceful fans, but also a few rowdies. That alone would be unfavorable enough for us, but on top of it all, these signals stimulate our bacteria and make them more aggressive. We also know this scenario from concerts when things get quite heated. Some of these bacteria can even convert stress hormones into a stronger form, which further enhances the effect. Chronic stress not only makes a living being itself a little thinner-skinned, but also its intestinal mucosa.

But the whole thing is not a one-way street, because conversely, the intestinal flora itself also has an effect on personal stress sensitivity. How can this effect be proven?

One of the best ways to explore the mysterious symbiosis with our bacterial friends are mice without their own microbiome, which are bred especially for this research. If you transfer a certain mixture of microbes into their small mouse-intestines, you can make sure that the corresponding reactions are actually caused by the microbes and not by the mouse genes, the environment or by a special kind of food. These germ-free mice (gnotobiotic animals) seem to exhibit relatively peculiar and unnatural behavior and characteristics. One of these characteristics is an increased susceptibility to stress. It has been shown that gnotobiotic animals, when under pressure, produce a much higher amount of stress hormones than their normal conspecifics. However, if they are administered a healthy microbiota in the mouse childhood, the behavior of these mice normalizes. Unfortunately no improvement can be observed in adult mice, which is probably bad news for us humans, too [6]. There is this part of our life that we could not influence ourselves, and that ship has sailed.

Studies on stress during pregnancy show that the first years in particular have a decisive influence on our whole life, as does the time before birth. The microbiome of the stressed mother is subject to the same changes as just described, it changes its composition and becomes more aggressive. In this case, however, this does not only affect the mother herself. In addition to the microbiome of the intestine, the microbiome of the vagina is also affected by this change. During natural birth, the mother's microbiome is transferred to her child and "impregnates" the new creature with lactobacilli from the vagina and a colorful collection of bacteria from the intestine (we will not go into further details here). This sounds disgusting, but is very important for the infant, whose microbiome is now developing within three years on the basis of this starter culture. In the beginning, it is mainly lactobacilli that enable a perfect digestion of breast milk. However, these useful lactobacilli of all things are greatly reduced in the vagina of a stressed mother. The consequence is a higher susceptibility of the child to intestinal-brain diseases [21].

A microbe-friendly and stress-free lifestyle, especially during pregnancy, can therefore help to give the newborn baby the best possible start in life. But it is also good for everyone else to actively combat chronic stress. There are many good approaches for this.

1000 Revolutions per Minute in our Hamster Wheel

The list of things to do is long, and bad conscience is omnipresent. We have to get up at five in the morning, check WhatsApp messages, have a quick green smoothie and then go for a morning run, check WhatsApp messages, take a shower, put on the right clothes, check WhatsApp messages, style or shave, wake up kids, prepare healthy lunches, drive kids to school or toddler group, check WhatsApp messages, go back to the office, work eight hours, process WhatsApp messages, then go shopping, store food, do the office work at home, recharge the mobile phone and tablet, supervise homework, cook, eat, check WhatsApp messages, clean up, put the kids to bed, attend advanced training courses, watch the news (and feel bad about it), read something educational, check WhatsApp messages and then off to bed, quickly have sensational sex with your long-term partner and then (after a reasonable amount of cuddling) immediately fall into a deeply relaxed state and fall asleep to be fit again for the next day.

On the weekends we should do more sports (because now we have more time), clean up and clean the house, weed, dispose bulky waste, polish our car to a shine, clean the windows, repair the lawn mower, clean the basement, clear out the attic, go to the pedicure, go for a haircut, dye our hair, do something with the kids, invite friends, say something clever about world affairs, volunteer, go hiking or cycling, go to the theater, finally visit our aunt/grandmother/parents/parents-in-law, buy clothes, do our tax return and worm our dog.

In a two-week vacation, we have to spend a day packing our bags, spend another day on the plane (while we are cramped in the Economy-Class), take an educational tour, visit museums, cycle or hike, we must not forget to inform all our friends and acquaintances in real time on WhatsApp and Facebook about the status of the trip, buy some more stuff so that the cellar, which has just been cleared out, can be filled up again, pack the suitcases again, spend another day on the plane, wash the holiday clothes, take the suitcases back to the attic, make a photo book, paint the fence quickly and prepare for work again.

Are we Completely Nuts?

Why do we have the idea of having to do all this? Why do we immediately feel bad if we don't do it? Is it really our own desire to live so hectically and externally determined? Or is this wish possibly being fed to us daily by the media and advertising, using methods of professional brainwashing?

Consumption is the magic word. It is recommended to jog or take fitness courses, which admittedly makes sense. However, we don't get this advice because sport is healthy, but mainly because in the best case we need the latest Adidas sports shoes and the complete clothing set for the modern jogger, including a fitness bracelet and mobile phone holder for athletes. We should not just cook because it's simply fun, but because we can finally be sold a sinfully expensive Thermomix, which makes the relaxed standing in front of the stove and stirring unnecessary. More time for old-fashioned cooking would ultimately only deter us from further purchases. It is not us who benefit from this tactic, but the elite, who already own the whole world, but still want more. To make this possible, we run day after day in our hamster wheel, like crazy and without a break. And sooner or later we perish from it.

Much of the above is fun - no question. I love round trips, even if they are not relaxing in that sense. Other things are really no fun, but still have to be done, for example the daily housework or the tax return. But not all of them, and above all not always perfect. You can also sometimes take a more relaxed view of things. Sometimes you can also take things more relaxed. Just tell your friends after your holiday: I only relaxed at home. I was in the garden, took a few short walks, cooked myself something nice every now and then and read a really good book. We almost have a bad conscience to confess such a thing while everyone else is jetting around the world with child and dog. But the one or other jealous look rather says: "I would also like to take such a relaxing holiday once in a while".

For me, relaxation is closely linked to the reading of a good book, no matter whether the content is instructive, exciting or simply funny. I would like to recommend one of my books especially, since we are currently on the subject of mental stress. My friends gave it to me with a wink, as I am known as a notorious control freak and constant stress victim: "I don't have to do shit! The manifesto against guilt." by Tommy Jaud. Although the humorously portrayed wisdom of the protagonist Sean Brummel is not to be taken unconditionally seriously, it not only makes the reader smile but also makes him brood. The next time our you-must-monster whispers in our ears "You have to clean the kitchen cupboards", although they are actually still perfectly clean, we might just answer him cheekily: "I don't have to do shit!"

Realistic Expectations

Everlasting happiness, perfect beauty and indestructible health - according to advertising, all we have to do is spend enough money and finally make a real effort, then we can achieve all this. This is of course complete nonsense. Nevertheless, films, advertising and other media have such a strong effect on our easily influenced brains that reason says goodbye and we become slaves to ideals that we simply cannot achieve. Realistic expectations would be much better for us.

Happiness

We cannot always be happy, not even the greatest optimists among us (for me, as a rather pessimistic person, this is very comforting). Instead, everyone has their own personal level of happiness, on which happiness swings back and forth. Some people are simply always super happy. On a scale of 1 to 10, their level is perhaps an average of 8, but in particularly happy moments they reach 10, and in particularly unhappy moments they drop to a level of 5. These are the enviable people who win 50 bucks in radio shows and then squeal deafeningly for five minutes. With other people (which unfortunately include me) the level of happiness is set rather low. If we would win a million (so far pure theory), our heart makes a little sentence, we smile a little with joy and on this day we reach a happiness level of seven points. Even under the best circumstances we can never achieve more.

Happiness research currently assumes that there are two factors that determine this basic level. Our living conditions are part of it, but at least 50 percent of it is our genes that are responsible [22]. This is where it becomes particularly interesting again, because only a small part of the genes in our body is human, while a much larger proportion of genes is of microbiotic origin. If the genetically determined level of happiness were only related to our own genes, we would basically have no chance of positively influencing this part. However, it would be very surprising if our bacterial friends, who demonstrably influence our health and emotions, had no say in matters of happiness, of all things. Logically, happy bacteria should also be able to raise the genetically determined part of our personal happiness level. There will certainly be new and informative studies in this direction as well.

However, regardless of the base level, there are these swings up and down. Our own childhood, recent experiences, social interaction and such trivialities as the weather or a good or bad meal make our mood sway. The great art is to live with these fluctuations and our personal base level and to regard both as normal and not so important. We are more satisfied if we can simply accept the circumstances without constantly questioning whether this or that makes us happy and whether we shouldn't actually be a little happier overall. We don't always have to shine with happiness and joy, even if it feels nicer, the advertising claims it and our fellow human beings then like us better. Sometimes it is also okay to be sad or in a bad mood. This does not make us depression patients.

Health

Unfortunately, we have similar unrealistic expectations when it comes to health. Our unshakable belief in modern high-tech medicine awakens the illusory hope for permanent, perfect health. However, this claim cannot be fulfilled at all, not even and especially not in the present day. Compared to the past, only the nature of our diseases has actually changed.

Infections that only a few decades ago were a deadly threat have now atrophied into small annoyances. Physical ailments or even the most serious injuries can be cured surprisingly quickly and without complications with the help of surgery. The pharmacy has a huge assortment of pills, ointments and other remedies for almost every physical complaint. Plague, cholera, tuberculosis and other diseases that claimed millions of lives are only known in the western world from history books. Fortunately, infant mortality continues to fall worldwide, as the following two diagrams show.

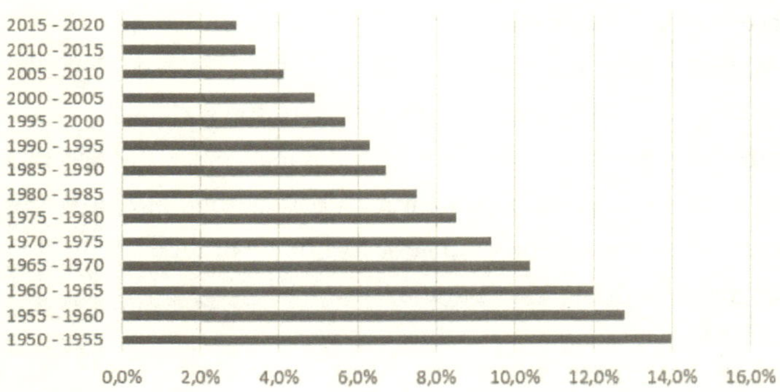

Source: https://population.un.org - United Nations, Department of Economic and Social Affairs, Population Division (2019). World Population Prospects 2019.

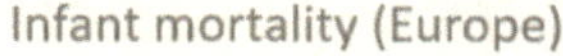

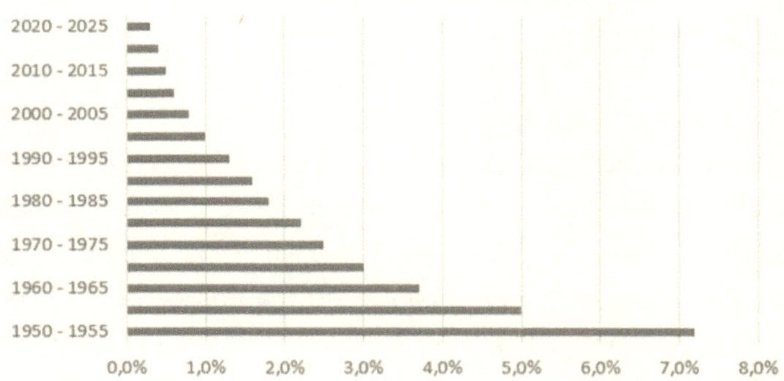

Source: https://population.un.org - United Nations, Department of Economic and Social Affairs, Population Division (2019). World Population Prospects 2019.

That's actually good news. Unfortunately, the western way of life has given us a lot of other diseases, so-called civilization diseases. Our modern epidemics are obesity, metabolic syndrome, diabetes, allergy, food intolerance, chronic inflammatory bowel disease, slipped disc, Alzheimer's and Parkinson's disease. Their triggers are lack of exercise, chronic stress, an inappropriate diet, harmful substances and a dwindling microbiome.

This is the world in which we must actually live and survive. We spend vast sums of money on drugs to relieve our sufferings. Most of the time, however, we only fight the symptoms of a disease without ever eliminating the cause. At the same time, taking these drugs triggers other problems, as the usually quite long list of side effects clearly shows. This way of fighting disease is extremely lucrative for the health industry - but deadly for us.

The change in our way of life cannot be reversed. The variety of different herbs, seeds, plants and animals in the diet of a Stone Age hunter has long since disappeared from our world and our diet. Most of our daily food consists of a few staple foods, such as wheat, rice, corn and potatoes. All the noise and stress of modern times is hard to avoid. Environmental toxins affect our health insidiously without us being aware of it.

Within this defined framework, however, we can optimize our way of life to avoid diseases of civilization. We already do a lot if we eat "real food", exercise as much as possible, avoid unnecessary stress and live relatively poison-free. The topic of living relaxed and poison-free also includes a certain acceptance of mild pain or diseases, however unpleasant they may be. Especially at an advanced age, when with every year of life a new ailment comes along and clings stubbornly to us. Not every bacillus in our body has to be bludgeoned down immediately with antibiotics. Those who are sick have no business at work (stuffed up to the neck with medication), but only in bed or on the couch, armed with tea and a hot water bottle - hero of the job or not.

Appearance

The perfect look is like the perfect lawn - both are almost unattainable and usually only achievable with a great deal of time and money, but even then usually only for a very short time. Nevertheless we are always unhappy about our appearance and our figure (not to talk about our lawn). In this case I have to limit "we" a bit. This issue seems to affect mainly women, while at the same time many men with the figure of Obelix feel like a kind of second George Clooney. Dear men, I envy you for this overly positive self-assessment! We women could use a lot more of that. Dear men, I envy you for this overly positive self-assessment! We women could use a lot more of that.

If there were no television, no magazines, no internet, no advertising and so on, we would only see the people around us and feel a little bit better. Unfortunately only a little bit, because with increasing age one unfortunately moves further and further away from the given ideals. This is probably not a modern phenomenon. A visitor of the Louvre is confronted in the sculpture department with numerous rather moderately attractive men in a higher age. But women over 30 were probably already unsexy in the sculptors of antiquity. Or the modelling of female wrinkles is simply too difficult...

Of course we're not stupid. We know deep inside that these ideals of beauty are nonsense, and that only a tiny percentage of humanity can even come close to achieving them. Even the most beautiful people in the world are additionally professionally made up, exclusively dressed and provided with a lot of soft focus before the public gets to see them. We know that we are the unlucky losers while all these corporations that sell us expensive products for "more beauty" are the laughing winners. And yet it gnaws at us every day.

On good days I stand in front of the mirror and think it could be worse, for my age I'm in pretty good shape. On other days I go through the list of cosmetic operations that I think I really need. Starting with liposuction on legs and upper arms, followed by a full body skin lift. After that, my terrible hooked nose would finally have to go, the nasolabial fold would bite the dust and a facial lift would dissolve my bulldog cheeks into nothing. Then there are the breasts, which could use a good lift, to be good enough for nude photos in case of doubt (if I would do any). A bit more chin would be nice too, then I wouldn't always look like a dolphin in profile. Finally, the many small skin imperfections and a whole bundle of daily growing spider veins could be removed. That's about how I would start. Probably a whole body transplant would be easier and cheaper, I am still waiting for suitable donors.

In moments of mental clarity, however, I ask myself if I am actually completely crazy to even think about all these surgical interventions. None of these shortcomings affect my health. Millions of women have thick thighs, cellulite and hooked noses. Millions of women have thick thighs, cellulite and hooked noses. Every cent spent means less freedom, and every surgical intervention poses a health risk, starting with antibiotic-resistant germs that lurk in hospitals and can lead to the amputation of a leg with even a small prick. Fortunately I am so thrifty, and fortunately there are those moments of mental clarity. Today's world offers many new possibilities. Some of them we can of course use to improve your personal quality of life and your self-esteem with little or no risk. On the whole, however, we should simply try to make friends with the circumstances.

Expectation is also the key to more satisfaction here. What can I realistically achieve with my inherited body, my age, the time I have left for sport and with a healthy diet? Would I really be so much happier if I were more beautiful or a few kilos lighter? It is known from happiness research that happiness does not last. Probably especially not when the expensive silicone breasts are purposefully moving towards the center of the earth again a year later. Instead of having all these unrealistic expectations, we should relax, do what we can and be satisfied with it. In the end we will not be perfect, but we will be optimally happy, healthy and beautiful. As soon as I have done that, I will write another book about it...

Learning to Switch Off

In our hectic world we have already reached this critical point, I'm afraid. We have indeed forgotten how to switch off. We can't help but always go full throttle, even when the concrete wall is already in sight. That's why it really helps to actively learn how to relax.

Yoga and Meditation

Everybody reads and hears about it, but very few try it out for themselves. But yoga and meditation really help.

Especially men seem to have their difficulties to get enthusiastic about such courses. But they should not! My employer offers (which I think is great!) health courses on the company premises. Instead of filling up your stomach in the hectic and noisy canteen at lunchtime, you can recharge your empty batteries at "Yoga at noon". There are actually some men in these groups who visibly feel comfortable there. So dare you, boys!

Yoga, in contrast to meditation, is a rather sporty approach. It is not only about relaxation and breathing techniques, but also about strength and balance. The teaching, which comes from India, also helps in case of doubt when lifting a big jug of beer (you may know the beer glasses at the Oktoberfest) and the subsequent somewhat shaky walk home!

Yoga also exists in a fun version, for example in our village: Yoga also exists in a fun version, for example in our village: The local brewery dream couple invited to the first "PReG" last year, which means "Pillmeier **Re**laxation Gymnastics". Of course I was there live and can therefore report. The event took place in the garden behind the brewery, and each participant received a half-liter glass beer, which was drunk as part of the exercise. The exercise program was created in the style of a Bavarian festival. The classic yoga figure of the "Warrior" was quickly renamed "Waiter", while the "downward-facing dog" became the "beer tent". We laughed a lot, but the one-handed "table" pose with a glass of beer in the other hand made some of us really sweat.

If you prefer a calmer way of relaxation, you should try meditation. You would not believe how difficult it can be to just breathe deeply and relaxed and not think about anything. The good thing is that both forms are very long-lasting. Once you have learned how to relax actively and consciously, you can use this technique anytime in your daily life. When driving a car (in which case please do not do it with your eyes closed), in the office or just at home on the sofa. Often we breathe all day long only flat and with shoulders lowered forward. Tense your shoulders, try to free your brain from all the thoughts that are buzzing around and take a few deep, conscious breaths - and the hamster wheel will already turn a little slower.

Let Yourself Relax

Yoga and meditation are active methods to relax. But there are also passive methods, which are of course more comfortable. These include wellness massages and other feel-good moments such as facials, foot care treatments, a bubble bath or whatever is good for you.

Massages do not exactly fall into the group of "bargains for the small purse". Unless you have a diligent partner with strong thumbs and some skill and empathy. But especially with this little anti-diet the money is well invested as long as the private budget can cope with such luxury spending. Otherwise you might be able to negotiate a small deal with your partner or a friend.

There is still an alternative to the strong thumbs of the partner and the expensive treatments at the professional. Office workers (especially those who additionally pursue their passion for writing at the weekend and after work) know the chronically tense neck and the painful area between the shoulder blades only too well. There is nothing more relaxing than when someone kneads these unpleasant tensions vigorously after a long day at work. Preferably as often as we like. Most of all, we wish all this without the obligatory half hour of begging before the massage and the famous moaning after three minutes of "Ouch, my thumbs hurt so much!". The electronic neck massager makes it possible.

I must confess, I would never have bought it on my own. Such devices usually end up in my mental drawer called "knick-knacks the world doesn't need." But this was one of the best gifts I've ever received. Quality has its price here too, but it's definitely worth the expense. With powerful circular movements, which feel as if they were made by a professional masseur, the machine kneads through the tense areas. These evening massages are small islands of relaxation.

Personal Time Out

You plan time for all kinds of things in life, at least if you're a little control freak and workaholic like me. The getting up, the work, the necessary shopping, the hated house cleaning, appointments with friends, and so on. The only thing that unfortunately always falls by the wayside is time for ourselves.

Maybe it's not a bad idea to consciously take some time off, instead of just hoping that one day all the work is finally done and we can rest afterwards.

I personally am a specialist in overestimating my own work performance. If someone who looks like me ever draws up realistic daily plans, this creature can very quickly be revealed as a shape-shifter or alien. My plans generally look something like this: I get up at 7 a.m. and bake fresh bread. After breakfast I could drive to the nature park (three hours drive there and back) and hike for a few hours, go shopping for food on the way back and then have the planned barbecue with friends in the evening. Reality was on that day: Fortunately, common sense made me cancel the hike. The shopping alone took two hours. I spent the rest of the day in the kitchen, preparing various salads, the barbecue and the most unsightly tiramisu the world has ever seen. By the way, this day was my birthday, and I still don't know the exact reason for the tiramisu disaster. Another classic of my personal planning history: " In the morning I will quickly paint the walls in the bedroom and in the afternoon I will lie down in a deck chair in the garden and read a good book." On that day, I was still standing in the bedroom at eight o'clock in the evening, with the paint roller in my hand.

For today I had planned to write until 15.00 and then read a book for two hours. Then I had planned to prepare my sourdough for tomorrow and then cook dinner. Actually I wanted to do the house cleaning in between. Now it's 3:11 pm, I will postpone the house cleaning until tomorrow, and now I switch off the PC and continue reading my thriller. See you soon!

Slight Movement

Sport is of course always good, but we are still in the chapter "Relax!" - and for that easy movement is more helpful than downhill cycling. We Bavarians like to live by the motto "the more, the better". Following this motto, I always thought that in order to be fit, I must definitely do the most strenuous sport of all.

There is of course a bit of truth in that. Sport - the disgusting, really exhausting sport with disgusting sweat and terribly aching muscles for the next two days - is unfortunately the only way I know to build up some muscles. But it is not ideal to go full throttle immediately. Several sore knees remind their owners for the rest of their lives. Especially in the beginning, but also between strenuous sports days, exercise without the risk of a heart attack is often the better alternative. Especially when it comes to the chapter on "Relax!"...

Then all you have to do is find out what you enjoy most (or at least what annoys you the least). One likes to hike through the woods with a backpack, the other may prefer to dance through life. Others may use the sweaty 35 degrees, which the summer sometimes brings, for a jump into the cool water. A walk in the surrounding area is also possible at any time, without much planning or expense.

All this is not only good for the body, but also helps the brain to shift down a gear. For example, when we concentrate on a steady stride and deep breathing and consciously perceive our surroundings while we go for a walk. By the way, moving the mouse, turning the pages of a book and zapping with a remote control do **not** count as "light movement", sorry!

Anti-Diet Part 2: Friendship with the Microbiome

Despite all the enthusiasm for the microbiome and its promising possibilities, we should be aware that the associated research is still in its infancy. There is still much to be done before we can say with certainty how the micro-biome and our body work together and what other influences are involved.

Eating with Pleasure – For the Microbiome

Despite several uncertainties, it is already definite that the greatest possible diversity of bacteria is essential for human health, and that a diet rich in fiber supports this diversity. Our diet is one of the levers we can use, while we have no influence on many other things such as environmental toxins, our first three years of life or our personal health history.

The principle of the Anti-Diet does not consist in compulsively following health rules. The aim is to support our microbiome with good food, fun in cooking and the love of fresh products in a very relaxed way. In order to achieve this goal, we should simply be a little bit open-minded and also include one or the other (real) food that has not been on the normal menu so far. You can try out different ways of preparation and combinations, but without any compulsion. You do not have to like everything just because it is healthy. Since 1890, parents have been trying to persuade their offspring to eat the hated spinach, although the allegedly phenomenal iron content later turned out to be a misanalysis. Spinach is tasty and, like any vegetable, contains many other useful nutrients, but the extremely high iron content was simply a hoax. However, we should rather not hope that one day science will classify fries, butter cream cakes and roasted pork knuckles as health-promoting...

The main component of a healthy diet - and almost all nutritional trends agree on this - is vegetables, pulses, fruit and wholemeal products. The latter have fallen somewhat into disrepute since the great wheat hysteria. However, as is so often the case, the question arises as to who benefits most from this general panic. After this enumeration, especially the vegetable refusers among us will surely have horrible pictures of unseasoned, semi-raw or only slightly steamed vegetables in mind. precisely here lies the problem.

A cheerful person who loves to eat and perhaps over time has accumulated a few pounds too many or has problems with the digestive system, decides to eat a healthier diet. He chooses one of these typical standard diets and usually starts "from next week". The formerly cheerful person spends the time before the dreaded start like the delinquent on death row, eats the last piece of cake and fatalistically consoles himself with the thought of a better life after the diet. After a few days, the dietary victim becomes sick at the sight of vegetables and surrenders to his fate with the thought: "I want to live healthy, but not if it has to be like this!"

Healthy food does not have to taste like feet. Well seasoned and refined with a little cheese, coconut milk or a dash of cream, it is still a vegetable, and it stays healthy. Even if vegetables are cooked a little too long and lose their vitamins, they still contain fiber. If the vegetables are spiced up with cheese or cream, the proportion of "possibly not so beneficial" ingredients, such as animal fats, is of course not zero. Nevertheless, it is demonstrably lower than for curry sausage with chips. Vegetables or even the boring lentils can suddenly taste surprisingly delicious with the right preparation. They automatically end up on the menu more often, because they taste good, not because "we should definitely eat more lentils". If it should turn out at some point that someone has once again miscalculated, as with the iron content of spinach, that doesn't matter much to us. Because in all this time we have done only one thing: we have eaten delicious food, and we have done it in a very relaxed way.

The reader, who has read the book description thoroughly before buying it, probably already suspects something. He will not expect a recipe list that is accurate to the gram and perfectly worked out as with the above mentioned standard diets. The Microbiome Anti-Diet does not prescribe how, what, when and how much to eat, because that would be completely nonsensical. As an author, I know neither the weight, nor the eating habits, nor the urge to move (or urge to lie down) of my readers. Two people who are holding this book in their hands right now certainly do not have the same daily routine or exactly the same preferences.

Most people feel comfortable when someone gives them very precise instructions. By nature we want to receive and follow clear rules to feel good and successful. Rule followed - topic checked off. This is probably one of the reasons why so many people put on weight again after a diet. In a diet with a strictly prescribed program, certain rules are followed for a certain period of time, but unfortunately the learning effect falls by the wayside. As soon as these rules disappear, we like to return to our old habits.

Most programs are also very complex and hardly compatible with full-time employment. They start with a very long shopping list and recipes where, for heaven's sake, you are not allowed to use the whole pepper, but only 87.5 grams of it. At least three times a day a meal should be prepared from as many exotic ingredients as possible. Most of them are usually only available in large cities or from some Ostrogothic indigenous tribes. For this reason alone, a certain relief spreads when the two-week Dr. Sebi diet (or any other diet) is over, the shopping list shrinks again and there are no 67.5 grams of leftover peppers in the refrigerator. Also, the regulations on the appropriate size of a meal cannot be applied across the board. Anyone who moves around a lot or has missed a meal is rightly hungry and can therefore enjoy a hearty meal without a guilty conscience.

Quantities stated in recipes of all kinds, even in quite normal non-diet recipes, are basically not bad. They give a good indication of the appropriate size of a meal, and it is quite helpful to follow them roughly. But it is even better to develop an inner feeling for satiety and amounts adapted to your own person. With the mountain of industrially processed food to which we have become accustomed, we have completely lost this feeling of satiety. We cook too much and then eat too much. On the side, we like to "snack" because everything is readily available at all times.

I am an absolute fan of Michael Pollan and his love for real food and simple principles. The following rule of thumb is very remarkable. "Eat all the junk food you want - as long as you cook it yourself.". [23] Mind you, it's a rule of thumb! Of course we do not produce everything we eat ourselves. Especially not our sweets. The only kisses I still get today are from Ferrero Rocher (delicious small chocolate pralines with a nut filling, called "kisses"). But the thought alone is helpful. Would I really eat a piece of cake now if I had to bake it myself? Or would I only eat it because I'm standing in the bakery and there are so many delicious cakes and tarts on display?

Quick Overview: Like or Dislike?

After much introduction we finally get to the point (hell, that took quite a long time). How do we continue with our Microbiome-Anti-Diet now?

We now hopefully have an idea of what a microbe-friendly and relaxed diet could look like and what the biggest problems of our western diet are. After all the writing I've done, I feel that I can demand a little more from my readers than just following rules - to be courageous, open and creative! I am actually not a Facebook fan, but I am a fan of the two short but meaningful keywords "like" and "dislike". That's why I use them for a small introduction to the Microbiome-Anti-Diet.

List of "Likes"

✓ Always think of Pareto. There's really no point in wanting everything to be perfect. Let's just leave the 20 percent of tasks that cause so much effort and instead put our energy into other important things.

✓ Learn to relax!

✓ Build up expertise in the area of food.

✓ Shop with respect for people, animals and the environment.

✓ Try something new (or even something very old that has been lost).

✓ Replace industrial products with real food.

✓ Eat according to your own rhythm of life.

✓ Experience satisfaction in choosing and cooking real food.

✓ Bring diversity into life with a healthy mix of fiber and vitamins for our bacteria friends.

✓ Bask in the feeling of success while enjoying a delicious meal made entirely without industrial products.

✓ Develop a little courage and a thirst for research to change a few old habits.

✓ Take the time to explore farmers' markets and other regional shopping opportunities in the area, instead of rushing through the usual supermarket and coming home with a mountain of plastic-packed stuff from New Zealand, Chile and India.

✓ Enhance your favorite dishes with vegetables and whole grain products.

✓ Now and then cook a little less than usual and additionally prepare a fresh salad or a portion of vegetables as a side dish.

✓ Allow the intestine sufficient time for automatic self-cleaning between the meals.

✓ Enjoy small sins without remorse.

✓ Move more, but with fun and lots of variety.

List of „Dislikes"

✓ Trying to lose weight at any price. Thinner is not necessarily healthier, often the opposite is true.

✓ Down with prohibitions! Everything may be eaten - with care and the consideration whether it can be spiced up with a few microbiome-friendly components.

✓ Compulsion. No one has to choke down something they're terrified of. However, when this horror extends to the whole range of vegetables, fruit and wholemeal products, it becomes a bit difficult.

✓ Stress. The package insert of Stress should clearly state: "Bad for the microbiome and deadly for its human".

✓ Compulsively regulated meals. If we eat less industrial food and thus less artificial appetizers, we will one day have a healthy feeling of hunger and satiety again. From that point on it is much smarter to eat only when we are really hungry. Or to skip a meal if we are still full. Consider rule number 57 by Michael Pollan: "If you're not hungry enough to eat an apple, you're not hungry."

✓ Getting discouraged! Our body is not a machine, but a kind of miracle. It is mysterious and enigmatic, and its reactions are often unpredictable. On the way to a new life with the microbiome we move forward, sideways or sometimes backwards. This is quite normal and no reason to throw in the towel (or even the fork).

✓ Low-carb pizza & Co. Yes, you can try them once - to satisfy your curiosity. Otherwise: If you want pizza, just eat pizza! Homemade, maybe even with wholemeal dough and vegetable topping, it is not as unhealthy as one might think. Even if you fancy a pizza in the restaurant - don't care about the calories and simply enjoy it! It's better to enjoy a real pizza every now and then (with delicious, fat cheese and all those evil carbohydrates) and save a few calories in the next few days, than to constantly desperately look for workarounds like the low-carb pizza that somehow doesn't make you happy in the end.

✓ Impatience. Yes, we all want to be healthy, happy and slim. And right now! But it won't work unless we run into the good fairy. Life is a learning process that only ends with death. Let's enjoy it!

These were very briefly the few basic principles of the Anti-Diet. Actually, it could start right now.

But without any idea and only equipped with a few likes and dislikes, the start is of course not easy. Therefore, here are a few details about the short tips, which you can follow in a relaxed manner and without any pressure, or not, or just from time to time. Where there are rules, there are always exceptions that haven't killed anybody yet (at least not immediately).

Down with "Eatremism"!

Yes, the word is spelled correctly, the spell checker has not failed here. I call the way food degenerates into a religion and a permanent topic of our time "Eatremism". Every year a new trend, it always has to be extreme, and in the forums there are fierce discussions and arguments whether you can eat this or that without losing the general certificate of the vegan/paleo-fan/low-carb follower.

Versatility is our strongest weapon in the fight for our health. We voluntarily put this weapon out of our hands when we ban entire food groups from our already limited menu just because they are not trendy.

Avoid Industrial Products

During the Anti-Diet (and actually forever, to be honest) we should avoid "edible food-like substances" (loosely based on Michael Pollan) as much as possible. In the beginning it is not easy, because many foods are not consciously perceived by us as industrial products. But as soon as we develop a greater sensitivity to the subject, we automatically produce more and more food and ingredients ourselves instead of buying them in the form of ready-made products.

The basic rules in Pollan's book "Don't eat anything your grandmother wouldn't have recognized as food" are a very good help to develop this new awareness [23]. This sentence applies to complete meals, but also to their ingredients. Now it is still necessary to find a relaxed middle course.

I personally cook more often than average and use fresh food. Nevertheless, my refrigerator and kitchen cabinets are still full of industrially manufactured products. Some of them are harmless, such as yogurt, cream cheese or my Thai curry paste, which only contains spices and ingredients that I would use anyway. But then there are such things as ketchup. I am fully aware that with the bottle of ketchup a pure sugar bomb is standing in front of me. But I eat it so seldom that from my point of view it is also okay. With other things, I read through the list of ingredients at some point and I am startled. I then try to make these foods myself or use them very rarely.

If the list of ingredients contains combinations of numbers and letters or unpronounceable words with a great many xes and epsilons, they are very likely to harm us and our bacteria friends. The approval of all this chemical stuff took place in a time before the discovery of the microbiome. There are about 320 additives approved in the European Union (EU) [24]. Most of these ingredients are added for more (artificial) taste, longer shelf life or a better consistency. Such additives are for example sweeteners, colorants, preservatives, antioxidants, acidifiers, emulsifiers, stabilizers or raising agents. Many of them may be used in unlimited quantities, with the small, non-binding recommendation to "add just as much additive as necessary to achieve the desired effect" (quantum satis).

In the EU, the European Food Safety Authority (EFSA) has been responsible for the health evaluation of additives since 2003. If we take a small critical look at the EU and the massive lobbying in its Parliament and the Commission, it very quickly becomes clear who in the EU actually decides which additive is supposedly safe and in what quantities it may be used. Some additives are rightly said to have an extremely harmful effect, which can be scientifically proven now that we are in the age of the microbiome.

Emulsifiers, for example, are used to achieve a better consistency of products. They are used to permanently bond two substances together. When mixing a homemade salad dressing, you have to whisk quite a long time to obtain a homogeneous liquid. If you leave the dressing in the kitchen for a longer time before adding it to the salad, the oil floats back up and we have created a kind of tequila sunrise of oil and vinegar. This would not have happened with emulsifiers. Unfortunately, even small amounts of these emulsifiers, far below the legally allowed amount, can damage our intestines.

Andrew Gewirtz's scientific team was able to prove that intestinal bacteria develop an unpleasant ability after absorbing a commercial amount of emulsifiers. They are able to overcome the protective mucus layer between bacteria and epithelial cells of the intestinal wall and thus promote subclinical inflammation, inflammatory bowel disease and obesity [25]. Interestingly, gnotobiotic animals, mice without their own microbiome, do not react to the emulsifiers administered. This clearly shows that the harmful effect is triggered by a negative influence on the microbiome.

Emulsifiers are contained in many industrially produced foods and do not have to be labelled in a generally understandable way. In Europe, for example, they are hidden behind numerous "E-numbers". These are codes for substances used as food additives, such as E322 (lecithin) or E472 (diacetyl tartaric acid glycerides). E472 is one of the emulsifiers that are approved for all foods and can be used without any maximum quantity restriction.

Emulsifiers are used, for example, in the following foodstuffs:

- ✓ Bread and bakery products (improved water-binding capacity of flour, kneading properties, pore formation and volume)

- ✓ Yogurt drinks (stabilization of protein particles for a creamy consistency)

- ✓ Margarine and deep-frying fats (stabilization of the structure for splash protection during heating)

- ✓ Chocolate (improvement of the flowability)

- ✓ Desserts (foaminess)

- ✓ Sauces (binding of fat and water)

- ✓ Low-fat products (creamy consistency)

Given this list, we obviously consume plenty of emulsifiers in the course of our lives. The best way to reduce the intake: Stay away from industrially processed foods whenever possible.

Artificial sweeteners are another example of harmful but widely used food additives. They are contained in many industrial products and are also widely used in private households as a sugar substitute to save calories. However, the health benefits have not been sufficiently proven, in contrast to the harmful effects, which range from metabolic syndrome (disorders in sugar metabolism, obesity, lipid metabolism disorders and high blood pressure) to the development of glucose intolerance. In the age of the microbiome, science knows more about the causes. The consumption of artificial sweeteners reduces the number of Bacteroides species in the intestine. The same effect leads to thin laboratory mice becoming fat. Under the influence of artificial sweeteners, the bacteria produce other metabolic products and supply their human with more extra calories in the form of short-chain fatty acids [26]. So we should be aware that if we try to lose weight through sweeteners, the shot will backfire.

Dietary Fiber - Crunchy Pleasure

Dietary fibers are the core of our Microbiome-Anti-Diet. However, as explained in the chapter "Winds of Change", these fibers can have some unpleasant and embarrassing side effects if you are not yet used to them. After my first experience with psyllium I could have told you a thing or two about it (but not without some annoying background noise). In that case, it is advisable to first reduce the fiber intake and patiently increase it gradually.

Our dietary fiber should come largely from vegetables and various legumes and to a lesser extent from cereals. This has nothing to do with the fear of gluten. The current hysteria about wheat and other cereals is certainly grossly exaggerated and mainly serves financial interests. Why earn just three euros for five pounds of wheat flour when the buyer also pays twelve euros for 500 grams of cassava flour (whatever it is)?

Nevertheless, there are reasons to reduce grain consumption somewhat. After all, it is very likely that our body is simply not prepared for the large quantities of cereal products that we consume with that much pleasure nowadays. Especially wheat, as the most widely used cereal, has been manipulated and over-bred over the years, which certainly contributes to its bad reputation. That is no reason, however, to strictly avoid all cereal products, even if one is suspicious of wheat in particular in the face of various campaigns. Unless you suffer from a medically recognized coeliac condition or gluten intolerance.

There are numerous alternatives to wheat, and we can use them as a substitute or in addition to bring more variety into our diet. But even then in moderation. However, you get used to not eating bread at every meal relatively quickly and turning the enjoyment of cakes, cookies & co from the rule to the delicious exception.

If we replace white flour with wholemeal flour and polished rice with natural rice, more food is left for our bacteria. To quote Goscinny and Uderzo, "Gaul is entirely occupied by the Romans. Well not entirely!" Again, Pareto applies. Again, Pareto applies. Foods such as tasty, crunchy baguettes also have a right to exist and really need not be demonized. Of course there are big differences here as well. "Good" baguettes are either baked by yourself or bought from a traditional baker. "Not so good" baguettes are sold in supermarkets as shrink-wrapped packages. Home-baked baguette contains: flour (optionally organic), water, yeast (<10g), salt. The baguette from Lieken (one of the leading bread and bakery product manufacturers in Germany) contains Wheat flour, water, salt, yeast, dextrose, E262 (sodium acetate).

Eat more Sugar!

There are no campaigns entitled "Eat more sugar". Probably because there is really no doubt that sugar is terribly unhealthy. On the other hand, although you can live without chocolate, cakes and delicious desserts, it's not worth it. But there are a number of things you can do to save at least some of the harmful sugar - without having to live like a Spartan.

A lot of sugar can be saved just by avoiding industrial products, because their ingredients follow a very absurd logic. Finished products that we would rather classify as hearty often contain large amounts of hidden sugar, while products that we use to satisfy our craving for sweets contain artificial sweeteners instead. We can also save an incredible amount of sugar when choosing beverages. It is not at all difficult to gradually reduce the sugar in coffee or tea and, above all, to do without sugary drinks such as lemonade, cola or even juices to a large extent. One gets used to it relatively quickly, especially with regard to the reward.

Thanks to the sugar saved, we can now and then treat ourselves without a guilty conscience to a delicious piece of chocolate cake, whose only health-promoting effect may be limited to the release of endorphin and dopamine. At this point, my friend Hans could give a little lecture on his endorphin theory, and he's probably not so wrong about that. If you doggedly give up everything and try to live 100 percent healthy, you are certainly not doing your health any favors. Because this strict renunciation means stress and we really do not want that.

That is why our Pareto goal is to reduce sugar wherever it is not absolutely necessary, especially in foods that should not actually contain sugar. For the desire for sweets: Better to enjoy sugar in moderation than sweetener in rough quantities.

Quality instead of Quantity for Steak and Chicken

We don't all have to become vegan, although PETA (People for the Ethical Treatment of Animals) would like to see that happen. Recently, the organisation has even been barbecuing fake dogs in public places to support this desire (which I find extremely tasteless, by the way, although I know what the eager ladies and gentlemen are getting at). Of course it would be nice if no animal had to suffer or die for us, but humanity simply hasn't got that far yet. We have been used to eating meat since we were small and it is difficult for most of us to do without it completely.

If a small fringe group becomes vegans, while the majority of humanity does not give the slightest thought to the living creature behind the piece of meat and only buys according to the motto "stinginess is cool", this does not really improve the overall situation of the animals of the world. Instead of going to extremes and splitting the population into vegans and non-vegans, we should simply all work together step by step towards "less meat consumption, species-appropriate husbandry and as little animal suffering as possible". Nobody in his right mind would want to do to a living being what happens daily all over the world in factory farming. Many people are unfortunately indifferent to this and do not even deal with it. This will not change overnight. Harari writes in his book "A brief history of mankind" about slavery in the past. People lived with it, not out of malice or hatred for the slaves, but simply out of indifference for their fate.

So indifference has a long tradition and is at the same time one of the worst human qualities. But even the publicly demonstrated and often instrumentalized mental torments of those who suffer with animals do not lead to any immediate progress. They are more likely to provoke resistance. I've really had all I can take of that current hype around the Veganism, although I cook often vegan and nourished myself for fourteen years meat-free. Everything and anything suddenly has to be vegan, from tofu (which by the way has always been vegan, even if it wasn't on the package before) to shopping bags. My shopping bags are not explicitly vegan and yet they are not made from the entrails of baby seals, but from cotton, jute or linen.

We need a healthy middle way, which will take us a step forward together and gradually convince more people of a more mindful and healthy lifestyle. There are two simple rules of thumb for eating meat. We do not have to eat meat every day or even several times a day. When we buy meat, we should look for the best possible quality, depending on our personal possibilities. For the welfare of the animals, but also for our own.

Only in this way can we all together show the agricultural industry that we no longer support their farming methods. Good meat can be recognized by the fact that it is not offered for just 3 euros per kilogram, even if the notorious bargain hunter's heart is beating faster at such prices. You can buy good meat at the butcher's, in the organic food store, at the farmers' market or even in the form of organic meat in the supermarket, depending on your personal account balance and logistical possibilities. The best thing to do is to take a little less of it in general and leave a little more room for vegetables on the plate, which is good for the animal world, the microbiome, the figure and also the wallet.

Nibbling

Frequent nibbling in between meals is not really beneficial (the diplomatic variant of "damn bad") because the intestine needs the breaks between meals for its cleansing. The migrating motor complex works for 90 to 120 minutes after the digestive process to completely cleanse the stomach and intestines. It stops immediately when new food reaches the stomach. If you feel like a piece of chocolate (and no one can blame you for that), it is better to enjoy it directly after a meal and let the intestine work in peace in between.

There is another argument against frequent snacks, namely the insulin level (with "s") and the subsequent release of inulin (this time without "s") to control the blood sugar level. Especially when eating sweets both rise and fall like on a roller coaster ride, keyword "insulin spike". This may sound exciting, but unfortunately insulin stimulates the absorption of glucose into our fat cells and the build-up of fat stores (storage lipids). The pancreas also has to work hard to produce enough inulin and to stem the insulin flood, just like the fire brigade does when a heavy rain has once again flooded half the city.

One can often read the advice to avoid "ravenous appetite" and rather eat several small meals spread over the day. However, if you take into account the issue of insulin levels and the self-cleaning of the intestines, frequent meals are rather counterproductive. We pay far too much attention to the stressor "hunger", perhaps out of boredom. A little hunger now and then does not hurt.

Low Fat Products

When we talk about healthy eating, sooner or later we get to the topic of fat. Body fat and fats in food. Both types are frowned upon by health fanatics. But both are there for a good reason. Fat in food is a flavor carrier and not per se unhealthy, and even our unloved body fat is very important for our health, as Giulia Enders explains in her inimitably relaxed way:

"Above all, our body fat makes us more organized. Without fat we would not be able to separate our cells from each other. This becomes apparent during anaesthesia, for example: The fatty cell membranes of the brain are probably made permeable by a mechanism similar to a flushing agent. The result: we faint. But fat is also a building block for stress or sex hormones, skin protection or even our fat deposits. If we lose too much weight, our internal organs can shift." [27]

Our organs should please stay where they belong, therefore: hands off low-fat food. Unless they are naturally low-fat, like chicken breast or cod. For just about everything else, the tasty variant with normal fat content is the better choice, but perhaps in smaller quantities. It was the anti-fat campaign of the 1970s that made many Americans and Europeans really fat, because the fat in low-fat products was replaced by another flavor carrier, namely sugar. In addition, there is the effect "If this stuff is low fat, it shouldn't be a problem if I eat more".

As is often the case, quality and quantity are decisive in warfare. The former is particularly important because fats are not filtered through the liver, but instead travel directly to the heart via the lymph vessels. A large amount of animal fats changes the microbiome and reduces beneficial bacteria such as Akkermansia, which has become famous as kind of a slimming bacteria. Therefore, it is a good approach not to eat fat in huge quantities, but to limit its consumption a little. But not by eating more artificial low-fat products! We want to eat with pleasure, and low-fat, tasteless fake cheese is the absolute opposite of pleasure!

Eating Less

Damn it. No one wants to hear that. I'll write it anyway. Smaller portions are the order of the day if we want to be healthy and slim. As hard as it is for us. Unfortunately, our brains are still living in the stone age and scream at us inwardly whenever we find something to eat: "Quick! Take as much as you can and eat it all!". Unfortunately, even after many thousands of years, our brains still don't know that nowadays we can find something edible every five minutes if we want to, and in huge quantities. These are far too often highly processed foods that easily suppress our sense of satiety.

I love food, and I always find it hard not to finish a plate. Especially since I usually put a lot of time and effort into the preparation. There is only one way to avoid the conflict: to cook smaller portions. When recooking recipes or cooking by feel, people often think that the portion is too small. But that is usually not true. The indicated quantities are completely sufficient.

Yes, it is annoying when half a can of beans or half a pepper is to be used. But both leftovers can be stored. Then you just have to be a little creative and use the leftovers in the next few days - often the best dishes are created this way. After all, we don't go on a diet with a fixed menu for the next three weeks, so there are plenty of ways to consume them.

A small incentive: If you haven't completely overeaten at mealtime, you can treat yourself to a bit of chocolate or a nice portion of nuts as dessert without a guilty conscience.

Superfood for the Microbiome

As soon as we become more involved with healthy and natural food, we suddenly like to read information that could be called "real food advertising". It is very interesting to see the huge amount of nutrients hidden in a simple carrot or apple. But at the same time, the greater knowledge about food and nutrients puts us in a quandary. We anxiously ask ourselves whether we really get enough of all the essential vitamins and minerals, not just from time to time, but daily or even with every single meal.

None of us really knows how much vitamin K is contained in our daily food and whether this amount is sufficient for us personally. That's why we suddenly find ourselves in front of a shelf with vitamin pills and as a precaution fill our shopping basket to the top. Michael Pollan calls this new ideology "nutritionism" - the tendency to break down the value of food to just a combination of scientifically identified nutrients.

We should definitely look at food as a whole and not as the mere sum of its parts. I completely agree with Mr. Pollan and am almost a little ashamed to have listed individual foods and their great properties on my website Mikrobiominfo.de. On the other hand, a little bit of advertising for real food may be necessary to put a counterweight on the other side of the scale - given the ubiquitous advertising for industrial products. While the industry, with various promises, packaging designers and psychologists, ensures that its products are bought and considered healthy (although they are not), the other side is left with only the appeal for "real food" and the modest reference to its numerous healthy ingredients.

One of these components are probiotics. Since we primarily want to build up our microbiome, they are actually the most important of all in this context.

Feed the Microbes

Our microbiome is only robust and healthy if we provide it with sufficient food in the form of dietary fiber. Therefore, this vital bacteria-food is of course one of the building blocks of our Anti-Diet.

There are different types of fiber, with different properties. Very special dietary fibers, called prebiotics (for example inulin, oligofructose and resistant starch), are especially interesting for us in connection with our microbiome. They have a particularly growth-promoting effect on bifidobacteria. Even an infant absorbs these bacteria with its mother's milk to build up its microbiome and immune system. They will accompany her or him throughout the entire life.

Prebiotics support especially the "good" bacteria, which become stronger and multiply more frequently with a rich food supply. This automatically inhibits the growth of harmful bacteria, because other harmful microorganisms and pathogens cannot settle in the intestine due to lack of space. It's like at a big party - you occupy a table with all your best friends and dearest relatives, so that the grumpy great-uncle can only sit down at the neighboring table.

The dietary fiber inulin is found, for example, in Jerusalem artichokes, chicory, garlic, onions, leek, asparagus, artichokes, black salsify, wheat bran, endive salad, parsnips, rye and bananas. Rye, oats, onions, garlic, bananas, tomatoes and asparagus have a high oligofructose content. Resistant starch is taken up with cold potatoes (potato salad), cold rice (sushi), white and green beans, kidney beans, wholemeal oat bread, green bananas and almonds.

This does not mean, however, that we should only focus on these few foods. Our bacteria friends are happy if we include them more often in our diet, but all other vegetables have many positive properties as well. If our daily food has a fairly high proportion of vegetables, legumes and whole grains, we can't really do too much wrong.

Of Cucumber Peel and Seeds

Though – there is a little something, perhaps. Here comes a quick plea to the cucumber peelers among us hobby cooks. Most of my friends and relatives are cucumber peelers (I hope they will not hold this paragraph against me). The poor cucumber will have its beautiful and vitamin-rich dress, and with it a part of its fiber, brutally torn from its body, before it ends up as a lifeless light green heap in the salad bowl.

I cannot fully comprehend this cruel act, but it is probably historically conditioned. In former times there were not these beautiful, slim, dark green salad cucumbers, but only quite profane chubby garden cucumbers with spines and rough, firm skin. Peeling is fully justified when preparing this type of cucumber, otherwise eating it is like a hearty bite into a cactus. However, peeling is not necessary with the conventional dark green cucumbers. On the contrary, the salad looks nicer, is crispier and above all has a slightly higher nutritional value. If the cucumber is organically grown, you need not be afraid of toxic pesticides on your food.

Other components such as seeds, dark green parts (in the case of leeks and spring onions) or membranes are all too often wrongly classified as undesirable and end up in the waste. As with whole grains, it is not necessarily the best idea to use only the soft interior and throw away the rest.

Sometimes there really is no way around peeling, as with white asparagus for example. I can tell you this from experience, because I once cooked white asparagus unpeeled out of stupidity.

If that happens, you can only bite off the tips and throw the rest away. Finally, there are also these certain things, which are certainly healthy, but with which one cannot befriend even with the best will in the world. In my case it's grape seeds, this bitter crunch when eating a sweet grape. I simply can't acquire a taste for it, no matter how healthy the seeds are.

But other things you should just try again and again. At some point, you will probably find that the fibrous parts or the many seeds no longer bother you at all or even taste better. We should then simply nibble our way through these different seeds, skins and membranes with pleasure.

New Friends for the Microbiome: Probiotics

Sometimes you can get quite lost in the jungle of terms. Prebiotics, antibiotics, probiotics, what are all these "biotics" actually doing?

Prebiotics as dietary fibers and bacterial food we have come to know a little bit better. Unfortunately, antibiotics are well known to us even without further explanation. Nowadays you can hardly find a three-year-old child who has not already been treated with antibiotics. And then there are the probiotics. Most people know from advertising that probiotics have something to do with yogurt and should be healthy. In fact, probiotics have a great potential, which is increasingly recognized by the industry. That is why they deserve a long chapter.

Probiotics are living microorganisms. They are added to many foods for the purpose of fermentation (conversion of biological material by microorganisms) or are already contained in the original ingredients. Additionally, they can be purchased in capsule and powder form. Some say that Probiotics are a good way to support the microbiome. Others take the view that they are either of no use at all or even cause harm. Now we need some good advice. Should we eat as many probiotics as possible, simply ignore them or even avoid them as much as possible?

Probiotics as a Remedy

Intestinal bacteria as a remedy are of course primarily suitable for intestinal diseases. There are always studies on curing various intestinal diseases with the help of probiotics. The results are rather mixed. Many of these studies end with measurable, positive results. Others hardly notice any effects.

Most of the positive results were achieved in patients with infectious diseases and colon cancer. For example, in a large-scale study lasting 12 years and involving 45,000 Italian participants, regular consumption of simple yogurt significantly reduced the rate of colorectal cancer.

Immunotherapy is another interesting approach in the fight against cancer and initially has nothing to do with probiotics. It is based on a targeted stimulation or suppression of the immune system to help the body detect and fight cancer. The success rate of this promising approach is still relatively low and science is currently trying to find out why. A healthy microbiome might well play a role in this process, as it can apparently enhance the effect of this cancer immunotherapy [28]. Again, the big challenge is to better understand the microbiome and find good strategies to support it. It is possible that one day there will be very specific probiotics to accompany immunotherapy.

Another interesting current research project is taking place in the countryside, this time it is not about the fight against cancer but about allergies and asthma. According to statistics, children who grow up on a farm are less affected by both than other children. Prof. Dr. Erika von Mutius tries to get to the bottom of the cause.

The environmental microbiome plays a major role in immunization, because on the farm, children come into abundant contact with a healthy and diverse microbiome by inhaling hay and straw fibers in the barn. The second part, however, again concerns the food ingested. It turned out that the protection was partly due to the consumption of raw milk, which still contains all lactic acid bacteria.

In a study that began in 2019, infants are given raw milk under controlled conditions. The results will certainly be exciting. Asthma prevention through regular drinking of raw milk – wow! Wouldn't it be great if asthma and allergies could be prevented in childhood with such simple means? Certainly not for the manufacturer of my super expensive asthma medication, but certainly for mankind.

Slim and Happy with Probiotics?

The fact that the intake of probiotics has an effect on the intestinal microbiome has now been largely proven. Only the specific influence of this effect on humans cannot yet be precisely determined. However, the statements about the exact nature of this adaptation of the microbiome still drift somewhat apart.

The composition of the bacteria in our intestine apparently changes both with a change in diet and with the intake of probiotics. However, this does not mean that new species of bacteria are being added, but rather that there is a shift in the quantities of existing species. This sounds somewhat unspectacular, but it is not.

This quantity distribution is closely related to the figure of the host of the bacteria. For example, Firmicutes species predominate in the intestines of overweight people, while Bacteroides are greatly reduced. According to a recent study, the same shift is also found in the bacterial community in the mouth. The oral bacterial composition can be used to determine the potential for obesity in young children [29]. So it is only this shift between the groups of bacteria that decides whether a person has to book one or two seats on the plane for himself. Or vice versa - perhaps overweight and the associated diet are the trigger for this shift, that is still the big mystery. However, various experiments with mice have shown that it is possible to transfer a "chubby" microbiome to slim mice and thus turn them into chubby mice.

The effect of these different sized groupings is not only limited to the body, but also affects our psyche. Studies have shown that as the microbial community changes, so do the signal molecules with which the microbiome sends messages to the brain. It is possible that a large part of our emotions and decisions actually originate in the intestine. Whether and how exactly this change affects physical and mental health is still an open question. However, this does not necessarily mean that this connection does not exist. It is very difficult to trace a specific effect of probiotics or even a change in diet because too many other factors are involved.

Probiotics in Food - Superheroes in an Acid Bath

In summary, we do not yet know one hundred percent what probiotics do. The effectiveness varies from person to person. There is no absolute guarantee of a positive effect. Therefore, one could well doubt that probiotics are beneficial to our health. Especially if they are taken in with food, for example with a cup of yogurt. The living bacteria in yogurt do not, of course, enter the large intestine directly (please banish all eventually emerging ideas about colon-yogurt-therapies from your mind), but have to take a detour through the entire digestive system.

The yogurt bacteria still feel quite comfortable in the mouth before they whiz rollercoaster-like through the oesophagus. But then things get dicey. Our probiotics end up in the stomach. As soon as they see food, cells of the stomach lining produce gastric juice, which consists partly of hydrochloric acid.

We need gastric juice to properly crush the food we eat, whether we have chewed thoroughly or gobbled down our food hastily. Another important task is to kill off pathogens and viruses. The stomach acid does both by breaking down all protein structures across the board. Unfortunately, this not only affects food and pathogens, but also our friendly bacteria. Most of them are attacked and killed by the gastric acid. Only a few superheroes survive, which is good news on the one hand. On the other hand not all superheroes are good, we already know that from the Marvel comics.

It's like always in life: The good guys are less visible, while the bad guys are more persistent. If our food contains harmful bacteria, the subsequent food poisoning shows all too clearly that even these few survivors can have a pretty evil effect. The poisoning is extremely unpleasant and in the worst case can even end in death. Most people will probably still remember the EHEC infections of 2011 with horror. EHEC is a specific strain of Escherichia coli bacteria, and they were ingested by the victims with their food. So all bacteria in the stomach are never killed, and the few survivors obviously have an effect on our health - in this case a fatal one. If this principle applies to harmful bacteria, it would be very surprising if it were not also applicable to beneficial bacteria. This is where probiotics come in.

Fermented Food

Fermentation is used to preserve food, produce flavors or break down tannins, without the use of preservatives or flavor enhancers. Yogurt, cheese, buttermilk, kefir and sauerkraut are fermented foods that we have all known for decades. A few new, exotic ones have been added by globalization, such as Kimchi, where my grandmother would ask "Kim...whaaaaat? Fermented vegetables even have two superpowers: they're prebiotic and probiotic!

Fermented foods are eaten all over the world and have a long tradition in many cultures. However, their health benefits were not the primary reason for their production. The original purpose of fermentation was to store food, in large quantities and without a refrigerator. How does fermentation help?

One of the many cool properties of bacteria is the production of lactic and acetic acid, which you can clearly taste in fermented foods. This acidic environment scares away putrefactive bacteria and thus makes food last longer. This was vital, for example, on a long voyage by ship in the days of the discoverers and conquerors. Before the 19th century, the most common cause of death among seafarers was not the dangerous voyage itself, but scurvy, and it wiped out entire crews. At that time nobody knew that scurvy was caused by a lack of vitamin C. James Cook was the first captain to rely on citrus fruits and the extremely vitamin C-rich sauerkraut and thus brought his crew safely to their destination. The good old sauerkraut could be kept on the ship for weeks because it was fermented and thus preserved. The smell on Cook's ship was probably less refreshing, but what do you do to live?

Although, from a purely scientific point of view, there may not yet be the ultimate "Go!" for probiotics, the personal experience of many people worldwide shows that the consumption of fermented foods has positive effects. It is precisely this long tradition of fermented foods that science is making use of in its studies. There is no simpler and cheaper way to conduct a long-term study over decades than to simply investigate the consequences of behavior or eating habits that have been common for many decades in a large part of the population anyway. At the same time, you can be sure that the people studied have not changed their habits during the period under study, influenced by their participation in the study.

Ilya Metschnikov, a Ukrainian microbiologist, made the following discovery. He noticed that Bulgarian farmers who ate a lot of yogurt and drank sour milk were extremely healthy and at the same time grew particularly old. The species of bacteria discovered at that time, Lactobacillus bulgaricus, was identified as the cause of these positive effects and is therefore still used today to produce yogurt.

Just in case you now feel that you have to put the book away to buy a pallet of probiotic yogurt right away: Every yogurt is probiotic per se. It does not do any harm, of course, but actually it is not necessary to buy a particular (and particularly expensive) "probiotic yogurt". Foodwatch has therefore been at loggerheads with Danone for years, as Danone's advertising strategy is based on attributing quasi-medical healing powers to its products such as Aktivia & Co [30]. The only important thing about a healthy yogurt is that it is still yogurt and not one of those sugary, artificial products enriched with artificial flavors.

There are also foods that have been created with the help of bacteria and fermentation and yet are not probiotics, for example rye bread. Sourdough, which is used to make bread, is produced with the help of microorganisms. Their gases create holes in the crumb and make the bread fluffy. Especially in the case of sourdough, the work of lactic acid bacteria can also be observed excellently in the private household, without the use of a microscope. No matter how many times I have done this, I am always fascinated when a mortar-like mixture of water, flour and the starter (which is simply a remainder of sourdough) has magically transformed into an airy, creamy mass the next morning. Unfortunately, the microorganisms responsible for this die a cruel death when baking the bread. If, on the other hand, we eat a fork of raw sauerkraut or kimchi, we also ingest a whole host of living bacteria at the same time, and it is precisely this characteristic that distinguishes fermented foods.

However, the bacteria in fermented foods do not travel through our bodies as comfortably and safely as their encapsulated counterparts. They are strongly decimated by the acid bath in the stomach. As soon as fermented foods are heated, the probiotic effect disappears. Sauerkraut can only develop its full effect if it is eaten raw, for example as a salad. As a Bavarian classic, namely the warm side dish for roast pork, it is still a healthy and tasty side dish with lots of fiber. However, the bacteria it contains have long since died during cooking.

Probiotics in Capsule or Powder Form

Harmful bacteria were always a problem, especially during historical wars. The hygienic conditions on site were extremely poor, and diseases such as typhoid, cholera and bacterial dysentery (shigellosis) spread and actually claimed more victims than the wounds caused by acts of war.

This was also the case in the Balkan wars of 1912 and 1913, during which the medical scientist Alfred Nissle examined a very special soldier. This soldier was the only one in his troop who had been spared by a rampant shigellosis. During the examination Nissle discovered an interesting strain of E. coli in the man's intestine. Apparently these special bacteria had saved the soldier from the harmful shigellosis. Nissle gave this Escherichia coli strain its name and tested it in a self-experiment. Later he applied this therapy to patients and successfully fought not only Shigella but also Salmonella infections. For this purpose, he filled the living bacteria in gelatine capsules to protect them from being destroyed by stomach acid. This method is still used today. In 1917, Nissle secured a patent for a product called Mutaflor, which is still on sale today and contains the "Escherichia coli strain Nissle 1917".

In the meantime, there is a wide range of probiotic products, both in capsule and powder form. Before purchasing, please note the following: Probiotics are not yet classified as medicinal products and are therefore subject to different controls than medicinal products, namely the safety rules for food. There are not yet any official quality standards for probiotics in capsule or powder form. They can be found in the shops under the heading "food supplements" and are therefore unfortunately lumped together with the alleged miracle and remedies described above.

The benefit of probiotics in powder form is a matter of opinion. Like the bacteria in fermented foods, they must first pass through the stomach - an ordeal that few superheroes survive. The advantage of powder can be the specific selection of very specific types of bacteria and their larger numbers compared to sauerkraut and other probiotic foods. But precisely this selection could in turn be a disadvantage, because the greatest possible variety is always good, and we are more likely to find this in sauerkraut, since not all useful bacteria can be processed into powder while still alive. Moreover, a real foodstuff offers us many additional advantages that a powder does not have: Vitamins, fiber and above all - pleasure. Perhaps swallowing a probiotic powder has the same effect than a hearty bite into a delicious piece of raw milk cheese. In that case I would definitely prefer the cheese.

If the aim is to add as many living microorganisms as possible to one's own microbiome, then (in addition to the somewhat more radical but extremely effective stool transplantation) enteric-coated capsules are probably the most effective way. There are now a lot of these capsules, from different manufacturers and with different compositions of bacteria. If many different strains of bacteria are contained in one capsule, they could have certain synergy effects. However, only a tiny part of the intestinal bacteria can be cultivated outside the intestine and transported in capsules. A far greater part dies immediately outside the intestine, and another, certainly very large part of our microbiome has not yet been discovered and is therefore not contained in the capsules. So diversity does not necessarily have to be the selection criterion.

The microbiome of every person is different. This fact complicates not only scientific research, but also our own path to health. A certain mixture of bacteria that has an immediate positive effect in one person may have no effect at all in another, or may even harm a third person. That is why it is worth experimenting a little at the beginning until one of the products works. If you are unsure or scared, it is best to simply leave it alone and rely on something that has been tried and tested for thousands of years: Fermented foods.

The Conclusion: Probiotics are Healthy and Smoking will kill you?

Why is it that despite so many convincing results, it is still not possible to state with certainty that probiotics are generally an effective remedy?

The first reason may be that science has not been dealing with the microbiome and the effects of probiotics for very long. Microbiome research will definitely remain one of the most interesting areas of research and will continue to produce astonishing results in the coming years. We will certainly soon know more about the effects of probiotics.

The second reason is financial. At some point in the future, a person's microbiome could be analyzed during a health check and the patient could then be given a personalized bacteria cocktail. If it is lucrative enough for any large company to have the method developed. Currently, there is no reason to do so. At the moment, the industry earns billions by selling drugs, natural remedies and therapies to sick people. Of course, our employers like to complain about high failure rates and the corresponding costs - that's sort of their job. But let's face it, thanks to the greatly increased automation of all sorts of work processes, industry no longer needs masses of workers, so a few more or less available workers probably don't carry any weight. The costs of treating the sick are largely borne by ourselves, whether privately, through taxes or health insurance contributions. The latter are reliably increased by the insurance companies at the turn of the year, no matter how angry we crumple the paper with the settlement. The health insurance companies have no real interest in reducing costs as long as they can reduce benefits without hindrance and increase premiums at the same time. So there are few reasons for the rich and powerful of this world to work on something that will make humanity as a whole healthier. That is up to us.

The industry has long since discovered the sale of probiotics as a source of income with high potential, which is why more and more such products are coming onto the market. But since they are not classified as drugs, these probiotics can currently still be sold without proof of efficacy, which might dampen the industry's interest in financing expensive research.

The main reason for the lack of ultimate proof, however, is the complexity of our body, which makes all studies about our food and nutrition difficult. Each person is different from the other in many ways. We are just not as "standardized" as laboratory mice. As long as it is (fortunately) not yet allowed to clone humans and produce them on the assembly line, it is impossible to conduct a study on 100,000 humans with identical characteristics. The second problem is the individual lifestyle during the study. If a study takes very long, for example 30 years, many conditions can change over time. Participants in a control group with an unhealthy diet could unconsciously change their behavior during this time, replacing French fries with steamed carrots and thus falsify the results. Little fibs are the third problem. In general, study participants who document their eating habits themselves tend to be inaccurate and to engage in small fibs - sometimes deliberately, sometimes unconsciously.

Therefore, while such studies are important and interesting, their results should not be overestimated. As long as research cannot provide clear evidence, it is up to each individual to try different probiotics - or not. If someone finds sauerkraut disgusting (and many people do), it would be nonsensical to choke down three portions a day just because it is supposed to be so healthy. There are always good alternatives, so there is something for everyone.

The human organism alone is already a complicated system, but the incredible amount of different microorganisms living in and on us is even more complicated. While our own genes do not vary much from person to person, the genes of our microbiome are as individual as a fingerprint. It is therefore not surprising that bacteria ingested with food have a different effect on each person, which is not one hundred percent predictable. However, the same applies to everything else our body is confronted with, both internally and externally. Many foods are healthy or at least harmless for most of us, while a small percentage of people are allergic to them. A face cream that causes storms of enthusiasm in 99 shoppers leaves a skin that looks like pizza in the hundredth shopper.

The slightly older of us (don't worry, we're still cool) still remember times when Lucky Luke casually carried a cigarette in the corner of his mouth, cigarette advertising was allowed, and the sexy cowboy with the Marlboro sat cool on his horse and planted the association "smoking is freedom" in our brains. However, the advertising nonchalantly concealed the fact that smoking undoubtedly damages the body in many ways. Lung cancer is one of the few types of cancer whose origin can be very clearly identified. Nevertheless, there are exceptions, because not every body reacts in the same way. The former German Chancellor Schmidt is said to have smoked more than one million cigarettes in his life and still turned 96 years old.But considerably more people smoke far less and still die of bronchial carcinoma.

Only one thing can be said with certainty: There is nothing in the world (and there never will be) that is without exception healthy for every human being or automatically makes every human being a patient. Above all, this will not happen to the same extent and at the same speed with two different people. This also applies to probiotics. But based on past experience in combination with the widespread use of probiotic foods, it can be assumed that they have a positive effect on the majority of humanity.

Sometimes you don't need to know, how the Magic Trick works

Even if the ultimate proof is still missing, probiotics should not be relegated to the realm of esotericism. There are many studies that have proven a positive effect of probiotics. Without being able to say exactly what causes this effect and how the individual microorganisms interact with each other. Do the microbes in the intestines defend their territory and kill the intruders? Do the new bacteria occupy free spaces in the decimated microbiome and displace harmful microorganisms? Or do the bacteria in the intestine perhaps even steal useful genes from the newcomers? So far, nobody seems to know for sure. However, sometimes one does not need to know exactly how something works in order to use it.

I speak into my headset in my office in Regensburg, and my colleague in Kuala Lumpur hears me - wow! When we have a really crazy day, we add another colleague from the USA, who has to get up very early, while my colleague in Asia works a late shift. When Skype is not on strike, the three of us can chat as if we were in the same room. It's actually a real miracle, our voices whizzing through the wires and reaching the right person (and maybe some NSA recording devices) in the world-wide jumble of conversations on the other side of the globe, and everything still sounds like our original voices! Do my colleagues and I know exactly how this works? Hell, no! There was something about electric vibrations and stuff, but how do they finally vibrate from my office in Germany to Asia and at the same time to the USA, and how do they know which headset to arrive in? Still it works, and we can easily operate a phone or Skype without deeper knowledge and use the technology we don't understand.

It works similarly with bacteria. The first written references to "leavened bread" come from the Bible, hundreds of years before the discovery of bacteria, which are still responsible for the acidification and rising of bread dough today. Nobody knew then what exactly happened, and yet the power of the microbes was used to make bread. Probiotic foods have also enriched our diet for a long time. With this pragmatic application to millions of people and for centuries, no long-term study, however well and widely conducted, can compete.

Anti-Diet Part 3: Cooking for the Microbiome

In order to optimally support our intestinal bacteria, we need one thing above all: a lot of fiber. And this mainly in the form of vegetables. But it is not necessary to follow a strict diet, to starve and to buy exotic food. It's all much easier, more varied and with lots of fun when shopping and cooking.

The third part of our Anti-Diet contains examples and ideas for the first 30 days and more. This chapter provides an individual concept for a healthier life with lots of joy in eating. Stubbornly following rules is not part of this concept.

The Hour of Creativity:
Personalizing Recipes

A year has quite a lot of days, usually 365. Sometimes we might go to a restaurant or get invited, but there are still many days left where our microbiome wants to be pampered by us. Now we need some good advice. How do we get the many good recipes we need to eat varied and tasty food 365 days a year? If something looks really tasty, it is usually not healthy and therefore disqualifies. Is that really the case?

With the following tips, it is easy to give the Microbiome Anti-Diet a chance for 30 days. And who knows...

✓ Don't limit yourself! Choose recipes that make your mouth water. Then check out the ingredients. Can anything be added/leaved/replaced to make this delicious food just a little bit healthier?

✓ As a passionate meat eater: Find vegetarian recipes and just add some meat. Before the big vegetarian and vegan hype, vegetarians often had to put up with the reverse: You take a meat dish and just leave the meat out - horrible! But the other way round works very well. Instead of a piece of meat with a boring side dish you can easily conjure up an interesting and spicy vegetable dish with a little meat on the side - perfect!

✓ Adapt to the season. In summer, fresh salads and Mediterranean vegetables are simply delicious. In winter, on the other hand, a steaming stew (in German, Arabic or Asian varieties) tastes and warms you up, and root vegetables make their big entrance.

✓ Everyone has their own personal, most hated foods. Don't be put off if they appear in an otherwise great recipe. Just replace them with something else! The only vegetable I can't stand even is celery. I therefore often replace it in recipes with fennel, which I like very much.

Pep up your Favorite Dishes Individually

Each of us has a set of favorite dishes. My personal hodgepodge of dishes is huge, because I love food and the best kind of globalization takes place in my kitchen. Depending on my mood I cook Indian, Italian, Chinese, Thai, Japanese, German or Mexican. Of course I don't want to do without my many favored dishes, just because some of them are not exactly the nutritionist's best friend. Sometimes we simply have to treat ourselves to something not so particularly healthy, and without a guilty conscience. But there is also a good compromise between healthy or tasty. In many cases, we can easily turn our personal favored dishes into microbiome-friendly favored dishes to do something good for ourselves and our bacteria friends.

My cookbook "Dinner in the Dark - Cooking for the Microbiome" follows exactly this approach. It gives the reader a few simple ideas that anyone with a little talent for cooking can use to pep up their favorite meal.

✓ Use bran instead of breadcrumbs - this simple exchange is simply great for the intestine! It works for many recipes. Meatballs (meatballs) can be prepared with bran, for example. The breadcrumbs on casseroles can also be easily replaced with a bran coating.

✓ Replace breadcrumbs with sesame seeds! The trick can be applied to almost all breaded foods, and in this way chicken, pork or fish fillets get slightly more fiber and less carbohydrates.

✓ Wholemeal pasta and wholemeal rice provide a nice portion of fiber and can be combined with any sauce or side dish. This includes the full range of Italian and Asian dishes, from spaghetti puttanesca to Indian vegetable curry. By the way, organic shops even sell the delicious basmati and jasmine rice in its natural variation.

✓ Give me the vegetables! There's always a little bit of space for additional vegetable left in just about every dish. It only tastes boring if the dish has been prepared unlovingly and uncreatively. Goulash and other casseroles taste even better if you add a large portion of finely diced carrots, onions and leeks. Slow frying and repeated removal of the vegetable base not only gives the goulash an awesome taste, but also a beautiful, dark color, and all this without using the "magic dust with many chemicals", which is known as "ready-made spices". Larger cubes of parsnips, carrots and pumpkin can easily replace half the usual amount of meat and make the stew pot simply delicious - and microbiome-friendly.

✓ Bolognese sauce, freshly prepared, contains a high proportion of celery, carrots and tomatoes, in contrast to the ready-made alternative from the supermarket. This automatically reduces the amount of meat. The meat can of course also be replaced by tofu or lentils if you want to try a delicious vegetarian variation.

✓ Potatoes can be replaced by parsnips (for example in stews) or by Jerusalem artichokes (for example as oven vegetables). Both have more fiber and fewer calories, but still taste very yummy and just a little different.

Five Hacks for Unpopular Foods

Sometimes we reach for food that we know is not really good for us. But we lack the alternatives because we consider the healthy option just bland. Or we don't eat many vegetables at all because we only know them from grandma's kitchen and didn't like them when we were children. With a little creativity, one or the other solution can be found for this as well.

1. Water as a drink is not very popular with many people, I know. But it can easily be transformed into a delicious drink. Slices of untreated lemons, limes and cucumbers bring a fresh taste to the water. Squeezed lemongrass stalks are also great. A sprig of mint or basil adds even more pep to the whole thing. Delicious, original, cheeky, tasty - and completely without sugar or chemicals!

2. Many people know vegetable side dishes as boring little heaps of steamed vegetables on the edge of the plate, which are graciously tolerated, but usually not eaten with pleasure. Enough with the boredom! Turn the vegetables in a little butter, together with garlic (finely diced or as a halved clove) and a few fresh or dried herbs such as rosemary or thyme or small cubes of pickled tomatoes. A small shot of high quality olive oil also gives a delicious taste. However, cold-pressed oil should only be drizzled over the vegetables after frying or steaming in order to preserve their valuable ingredients.

3. Kohlrabi is quite wrongly considered one of the rather unpopular vegetable varieties. It tastes really delicious and is still quite healthy if you steam it with a small shot of white wine, some cream and a lot of garlic. For an even more interesting look and taste you can add its leaves cut into strips. The result is a tasty side dish that could convince even kohlrabi-haters. A small cube of blue cheese makes it even more delicious - but you should make sure that you use more kohlrabi than cream and cheese.

4. Cauliflower tastes great with a sauce made from curry and coconut milk. Again, you should be able to still see the cauliflower in the sauce - so don't overdo it with the coconut milk!

5. If you can't quite get used to the typical kind of spinach, you might prefer the spicier Kurdish version. Tomato paste, cinnamon, cumin and coriander give the Kurdish spinach a touch of exoticism.

Three Great Recipes from Cookbooks

I love cookbooks! When I plan my meal for the coming week, I often sit down on the couch armed with a stack of cookbooks and leaf through them according to delicious recipes. The following recipes are from some of my cookbook favorites. Small adjustments make it easier to prepare these delicious dishes even after a long day at work or to support our bacteria friends a little bit more. The listed recipes are such variations, the source with the original is always included.

Tuna Casserole with White Beans

A recipe from a very old cookbook, rediscovered last year - sometimes you can find such treasures. The picture does not look very attractive in the cookbook, but the casserole tastes simply delicious!

Source: Das große Buch der Fische & Meeresfrüchte (The great book of fish & seafood), Könemann, ISBN 3-8290-3998-0, p.259

Variation for microbe friends with little time:

✓ For an uncomplicated preparation after work I use canned beans instead of dried ones.

✓ Depending on preference and availability, white giant beans or small white beans can be used. However, smaller beans give the casserole a slightly softer consistency.

✓ The dose of onions, garlic and herbs is higher in my modified recipe - herbs are actually never too much, are they?

✓ The fresh thyme can of course also be replaced by dried thyme.

✓ As an extra vegetable portion I add one carrot and half a stick of leek per person.

✓ Fish stock gives the casserole an even fishier flavor, but is relatively expensive and not always easily available, which is why I often replace it with vegetable stock.

✓ I replace the breadcrumbs with bran and thus provide my bacteria with an extra portion of healthy food.

✓ I usually replace butter with olive oil.

✓ Since I rarely cook for six people, in my variant the quantities are given for two hungry people.

Ingredients (variation, 2 persons)

    1 tin of white beans, 400 g
    2 tablespoons olive oil
    1 red onion, chopped
    2 cloves of garlic, chopped
    2 carrots, cut into cubes
    1 stick of leeks, sliced
    2 tsp coriander, ground
    1 tsp finely grated lemon peel
    2 tsp thyme (fresh or dried)
    150 ml white wine
    150 ml fish stock or vegetable stock
    1 can of tuna, drained
    plenty of basil leaves
    2-3 large tomatoes, cut into thick slices

For the topping:

    Two handfuls of bran (oats, wheat, ...)
    2 cloves of garlic, chopped
    1 bunch fresh parsley, finely chopped
    A shot of olive oil

Preparation (variation)

Drain the beans. Preheat the oven to 210 °C (410°F).

Heat some oil in a medium sized pot. Sauté onion, garlic, coriander, lemon peel and thyme over medium heat for 5 minutes. Add the carrots and leeks and continue to fry for 5 minutes. Put the vegetables aside on a plate.

Add the white wine and stock to the pot and reduce the liquid to about half at high heat. Add the beans to the pot and heat up over medium heat. Add the vegetables again and mix everything well.

Pour the bean mixture into the casserole. Cover with tuna, basil and tomatoes.

Mix the bran, garlic and parsley for the topping. Pour over the tomatoes, drizzle with olive oil and bake for 30 minutes until the crust is golden brown.

"Mixed Forces" Plate

My favorite dish from the books of Hildmann, also for non-vegans a culinary delight. The original recipe is basically perfect as it is, so my variation contains only minimal adjustments.

Source: Vegan for Fit (Attila Hildmann), Becker Joest Volk Verlag, ISBN 978-3-938100-81-3, p. 153

Variation for garlic fans:

- ✓ Since I love garlic, an extra clove refines the hummus.

- ✓ I personally do not use herbal salt, I prefer to use normal salt and fresh herbs.

- ✓ 1 broccoli is perfectly adequate, except when it is tiny, in which case you can take two (Attila takes 2 in his recipe, but nobody can eat that much broccoli!).

- ✓ I steam the broccoli instead of cooking it in boiling water to preserve the vitamins.

- ✓ The use of mineral water for cooking is an Attila special, in my case the water from the tap does it perfectly.

- ✓ Tahini (a paste made from sesame seeds) is per se not available in every village supermarket and once opened, it does not last forever. It is not worth buying dark tahini especially for this recipe - light tahini does the same.

The preparation remains the same - but I grill the vegetables on medium level instead of baking them at 250° C (482°F). It then remains a bit more firm to the bite.

Ingredients (variation, 2 persons)

For the "Mixed Forces" Plate:
600 g Hokkaido pumpkin
1 tsp paprika
Salt
Approx. 7 tablespoons of olive oil
1 garlic clove
½ - 1 eggplant
1 broccoli
1 tablespoon lemon juice
Salt
30 g sunflower seeds

For the hummus:

200 g cooked chick peas
30 g Tahini
1 tablespoon lemon juice
1 tsp ground cumin
½ tsp salt
40 ml cold water
1-2 garlic cloves

Additionally:

1 chili pepper
¼ bunch of flat parsley
½ tsp paprika

Preparation (variation)

Preheat oven grill to medium heat.

Wash the pumpkin, cut it in half and remove the seeds. Cut the pumpkin with a sharp knife into narrow slices. Mix with paprika powder, sea salt and 2 tablespoons olive oil.

For the eggplant, peel and finely chop the clove of garlic. Wash and slice the eggplant Season with a mixture of 2 tablespoons of olive oil, garlic and sea salt. Spread the pumpkin and eggplant evenly on a baking tray covered with aluminium foil. Grill in the oven on the top shelf for about 15-17 minutes.

Wash the broccoli and cut approx. 500 g florets from the stalk. Steam over boiling salt water for about 3-5 minutes. Drain in a sieve. Mix carefully with 2 tbsp. olive oil, lemon juice, herb salt and sunflower seeds.

For the hummus, puree all ingredients in a blender.
Wash the chili pepper and cut into fine rings. Wash parsley, shake dry and chop finely.

Spread hummus in the middle of two plates. Dust with paprika powder and sprinkle with chopped parsley and a dash of olive oil. Arrange the pumpkin, broccoli and eggplant around it. Garnish the eggplant with chili rings and some parsley.

Vegetable-Lentil Stew with Pan-Fried Feta

I have cooked this recipe so often that I actually don't need the book anymore. I love lentils anyway, but this recipe gives them a touch of sauce Bolognese, and the delicious feta is a dream! Again, no big changes are necessary - the recipe already contains plenty of fiber.

Source: Herbst, Winter, Gemüse! (Autumn, winter, vegetables!) (Cornelia Schinharl), Gräfe und Unzer Verlag, ISBN 978-3-8338-3438-7, p. 66

Variation for crunchy vegetables:

- ✓ The recipe is also converted here for 2 hungry persons

- ✓ Instead of yellow beets, I use carrots. In my opinion, they taste better than yellow beets.

- ✓ The cheese can also be coated with sesame seeds or bran.

- ✓ The preparation of the vegetables is described in great detail in the original recipe, so I shorten it considerably.

- ✓ However, I do not leave the vegetables in the pot with the lentils, but put them aside on a plate so that they remain a little crispy.

- ✓ Feta is simply delicious, which is why I always treat myself to a little more of it.

Ingredients (variation, 2 persons)

300 g carrots
150 g celeriac
1 medium thick leek stick
2 cloves of garlic
1 dried chili pepper
1 tsp dried thyme leaves
4 tablespoons of olive oil
150 g brown, black or green lentils
Approx. 300 ml mild vegetable stock
2 tsp tomato paste
1 tablespoon cider vinegar
salt / black pepper
1 tsp honey
200 g sheep's cheese (feta)
2 tablespoons sesame seeds or bran
1 tablespoon butter

Preparation (variation)

cut the carrots into about ½ cm, the celery into cubes of about 1
cm. Cut the leek into strips. Cut garlic and chili pepper into
slices.

Heat 2 tablespoons of oil in a pot and sauté the vegetables with
garlic, chili and thyme.
Put the vegetables aside on a plate.

Wash the lentils and put them in the pot. Pour in the broth and
cook covered over a low heat.
After about 15 minutes (the lentils should still be very firm to
the bite) add the vegetables to the lentils in the pot, heat briefly
on medium heat and simmer lightly for another 15 - 20 minutes
with the lid closed on a low heat. If necessary, add some more

stock. Season with salt, vinegar, tomato paste, pepper and honey.

In the meantime, cut the feta into 2 thin slices of the same size and turn in sesame seeds or bran.

Shortly before the end of the cooking time, fry the feta in a coated pan over high heat for about 1 minute on each side.

Arrange the vegetable stew with feta.

Favorite Recipes Online

In order to eat tasty, healthy and varied food, we do not have to reinvent the wheel or follow special diet plans. If we know what is important, we can find great recipes everywhere. There are incredibly professional food blogs and other recipe collections on the Internet. Many of these recipes are already very healthy anyway, others we can modify individually.

One-Pot

Also known as "stew." Stew is actually always good, especially in winter. Once the vegetables have been chopped, the rest is done by itself. In the meantime, the cook can do small jobs, read a little or do a quarter of an hour of yoga to relax the neck.

- ❖ **Cookie and Kate** - Chili sin Carne
  (https://cookieandkate.com/vegetarian-chili-recipe/)

- ❖ **HappyCarb** - Magic metabolism cabbage soup
  (https://happycarb.de/rezepte/suppen-eintoepfe/magic-stoffwechsel-kohlsuppe/)
  Unfortunately, the recipe is in German language, but you should really try it - the online translator will help you!

- ❖ **HappyCarb** - Fiery bean pot
  (https://happycarb.de/rezepte/suppen-eintoepfe/feuriger-bohnentopf/)
  The same here, it's in German, but so delicious that I couldn't replace it with something similar. It contains not only kidney beans but also green beans and is therefore something very special.

❖ **HeavenLynnHealthy** - Moroccan chickpeas, kale and sweet potato stew (https://www.heavenlynnhealthy.com/moroccan-spiced-chickpea-kale-and-sweet-potato-stew/)

❖ **Kitchenstories** – German-style leek and cheese soup (https://www.kitchenstories.com/en/recipes/german-style-leek-and-cheese-soup)

Super Bowls

Healthy recipes are often said to be bland and boring. Given the choice in restaurants and various slimming recipes, this opinion is perfectly understandable. But there is an awesome trend that proves the opposite: Bowls. I love them. Bowls are damn elaborate, but the result really speaks for itself. A beautiful bowl offers a colorful variety that can hardly be surpassed.

❖ **Platingsandpairings** - Sweet Potato & Chickpea Buddha Bowl (https://www.platingsandpairings.com/sweet-potato-chickpea-buddha-bowl/)

❖ **Fitfoodiefinds** – Kung Pao Buddha Bowls (https://fitfoodiefinds.com/vegetarian-kung-pao-quinoa-bowls/)

❖ **Foodheaven** – Roasted Chickpea Quinoa Bowl (https://foodheavenmadeeasy.com/roasted-chickpea-quinoa-salad-bowl/)

- ❖ **Wholeandheavenlyoven** – Greek Chicken and Quinoa Bowl
  (https://wholeandheavenlyoven.com/2018/01/15/meal-prep-greek-chicken-quinoa-bowls/)

- ❖ **cookieandkate** – Build-your-own Buddha Bowl
  (https://cookieandkate.com/buddha-bowl-recipe/)
  The instructions for the very creative ones!

Vegan Recipes

You don't have to be vegan to love vegan recipes. They usually have a big advantage called "vegetables". Plenty of vegetables! That's why they are always a good choice for meat eaters and vegetarians.

Animal fats are one of the ingredients which, especially in large quantities, have been shown to have a very negative effect on our microbiome. Too much animal fat in the diet promotes inflammation, which in turn promotes obesity, which in turn promotes inflammation, and so on. However, the question of what exactly "too much" means can be debated. But we do not want to make a religion out of it and we do not want to become perfectionists. A restriction of meat and other animal products certainly makes sense, but we don't have to convert to veganism.

There is nothing wrong with a varied mix of vegan, vegetarian and meat or fish meals. Even if vegans said "Fie!", a vegan meal can be wonderfully combined with some fish or meat and is then still much healthier than Mac and Cheese or a burger with fries. But many vegan dishes are so great that you really don't miss the meat.

- ❖ **Kitchenstories** - Hot chickpea soup (https://www.kitchenstories.com/en/recipes/hot-chickpea-soup)

- ❖ **cooktogether** - Steamed pak choi with ginger and garlic (https://cooktogether.com/recipe-items/steamed-pak-choi-with-ginger-and-garlic/)

- ❖ **skinnytaste** - Kung Pao Tofu (https://www.skinnytaste.com/kung-pao-tofu/)

- ❖ **spoonforkbacon** – Spicy Roasted Cauliflower over Hummus (https://www.spoonforkbacon.com/spicy-roasted-cauliflower-over-hummus/#wprm-recipe-container-17867)

- ❖ **earthyfeast** – Funky Green Tacos (http://www.earthyfeast.com/recipe/funky-green-tacos/)

- ❖ **feastingathome** – Crispy vegan quinoa cakes with tomato-chickpea relish (https://www.feastingathome.com/quinoa-cakes-with-cherry-tomato-mint-and-chick-pea-relish/)

- ❖ **feastingathome** – simple baked sheet-pan ratatouille! (https://www.feastingathome.com/quinoa-cakes-with-cherry-tomato-mint-and-chick-pea-relish/

Curries

There is nothing more delicious than a steaming curry, preferably nice and hot. The most important ingredient except lots of vegetables: spices, spices, spices. There are some nice spice mixes, for example Indian Madras curry or red Thai curry as paste. However, if you love curry, you may want to buy the necessary spices separately to create your own individual blends.

One of my favorite spice shops is Achterhof, a family-run business selling top quality spices. However, I am not sure if they also deliver abroad. But that doesn't matter, because in almost every country there are shops that sell high quality spices. It is definitely worth the expense!

You don't really need a recipe for curries. Just about everything we find in the house and garden can be used - carrots, zucchini from your own garden, half a pumpkin from the last meal. No matter what is in season or what is left over, you can certainly turn it into a great curry. If you want to compensate for a gourmet day, enjoy your curry pure. For the big hunger and more strength for the next hike there is delicious wholemeal basmati rice to go with it.

- ❖ **Bbcgoodfood** - Satay sweet potato curry
  (https://www.bbcgoodfood.com/recipes/satay-sweet-potato-curry)

- ❖ **Healthiersteps** - Turnip Curry
  (https://healthiersteps.com/recipe/turnip-curry/)

- ❖ **Cupfulofkale** - Creamy Cauliflower and Chickpea Curry (https://cupfulofkale.com/vegan-cauliflower-and-chickpea-curry/)

- ❖ **Minimalistbaker** - 30-Minute Coconut Curry (https://minimalistbaker.com/30-minute-coconut-curry/)

- ❖ **Jamieoliver** - Fantastic fish tikka curry (https://www.jamieoliver.com/recipes/fish-recipes/fantastic-fish-tikka-curry/)

- ❖ **Bbcgoodfood** – Spinach, sweet potato & lentil dhal (https://www.bbcgoodfood.com/recipes/spinach-sweet-potato-lentil-dhal)

Spontaneous-Dishes and Own Creations

Sometimes we have no time and no idea where we can quickly and spontaneously find a good recipe. Or we just don't feel like cooking with a recipe. There are many very simple dishes that, with a little experience in the kitchen, you can make without any recipe. At the same time, these own creations are wonderfully suitable for recycling leftovers - after all, we don't want to waste any food. Whatever the fridge or freezer can provide, there is certainly room for it in one of these spontaneous-dishes.

- ✓ Wholemeal pasta with tomato or cream sauce and extra vegetables in the sauce

- ✓ Salad with everything that is in season, looks delicious or must be used up (cheese cubes, tuna, salmon, tomatoes from the garden, half a cucumber from the vegetable drawer, olives, pumpkin seeds, sunflower seeds, chicken breast, ...)

✓ Chili Con/Sin Carne in all variations (optionally with whole grain baguette)

✓ Fish (e.g. cod-back fillet) with crispy Jerusalem artichoke and any seasonal vegetables

✓ Lentil stew with root vegetables

✓ Chicken or halloumi with vegetables from the oven, Mediterranean spiced

✓ Salmon steaks with salads (for example fennel and tomato salad)

✓ Meat or fish with sesame breading, roasted vegetables and salad

✓ Wraps, hot or cold stuffed (for example with rocket, avocado, carrots, tofu, kidney beans, coleslaw, falafel, peppers, tomatoes, pumpkin slices, ...)

Small Office Meals

Think unconventionally, be creative! In terms of "this is what a lunch must look like" we have adopted a certain pattern. We should break out of this prison very quickly! Instead of the usual sandwich with ham and cheese and a chocolate bar for dessert, we can take a mixture of fruit, vegetables, nuts, yogurt and many other delicious things to work, depending on the season. Sounds boring and elaborate, but it's not! All we need is a food storage container and a few ideas.

- ✓ strawberries, blueberries and a handful of Brazil nuts

- ✓ An apple and a cup of kefir or yogurt (my standard meal, because it is so easy to take with you)

- ✓ Yogurt with pineapple pieces, coconut flakes, honey and a few dried apricots

- ✓ One or two carrots, walnuts and prunes

- ✓ Cocktail tomatoes with basil and mozzarella balls, for dessert a few cherries

- ✓ Smoothie made from spinach, pineapple, banana and linseed

- ✓ Shake of berries and yogurt

- ✓ Yogurt with honey, coconut flakes, linseed and orange pieces

- ✓ Cucumber and carrot sticks with cream cheese, served with a handful of cashew nuts

- ✓ Carrot sticks or celery sticks (somebody will probably like them) with hummus

- ✓ Warm porridge made of oatmeal, water, cinnamon, honey, raisins and an apple (perfect in winter when fingers are cold in the office)

- ✓ Banana shake made from banana, buttermilk and linseed

- ✓ Pear with a piece of cheese and dried figs

- ✓ Cheese with grapes

✓ Kefir and mixed dried fruit (plums, apricots, mangoes, etc.)

✓ Yogurt with crunchy muesli and dried banana pieces

✓ Muesli with banana and mandarins

Here is a little additional tip: I have a small supply of nuts and dried fruit In my desk drawer in the office. If the hunger is greater than the meal I brought with me, I am happy about the small dessert. It often saves me from culinary folly.

3... 2... 1... Go!

Freshly inspired, we can actually start right now. The Microbiome Anti-Diet doesn't have to be elaborately planned or start on a Monday (just because that's the worst day of the week anyway). If today is Tuesday, there is no reason why we shouldn't start on Wednesday, or even immediately.

From the contents of the fridge you can certainly conjure up something delicious, as long as there is not just a bottle of champagne in it. Perhaps something edible is growing in the garden? Perfect! Reach out and create something that will make your mouth water.

If it is the weekend and you are invited somewhere tomorrow, don't worry. Go to the party, enjoy the good food and drinks, laugh with your friends and don't limit yourself! It's part of the diet and belongs to the category "Relax!".

Is the sun shining? Then just get your sneakers or hiking boots and get out into the fresh air! Unless you really don't feel like it right now, then just stay on the couch or in the garden and read a good book instead. Everything is compatible with the Anti-Diet. Have fun with it!

Afterword

Thank you very much for your brave perseverance until the end!

I hope the Anti-Diet has inspired you and helped you in one way or another. For example with new motivation or simply with some interesting insights. Maybe even with a smile or two about our completely crazy world.

A short note on the facts and figures in the book: As already mentioned, I am not a physician or microbiologist, but my knowledge comes from books and articles. Their data, for example about the number of bacteria in the intestine, often vary greatly. Nobody seems to really know exactly. Of course, I too have no way of finding out the only truth - perhaps it doesn't even exist. I collect information and draw my personal conclusions from it to the best of my knowledge and belief. Many of them have helped me a lot on my own way to better health, so I want to pass on this knowledge. I am constantly learning, and with the new knowledge I sometimes discard some earlier beliefs in order to remain open to new ones.

In some chapters of this book I have taken the liberty of copying from myself and used parts of my website (www.mikrobi-ominfo.de). If you find the microbiome as interesting as I do, please visit me there. I am very happy about every comment left, which helps me to improve the site and see what would interest you and other readers most.

Finally, I have a small request for you as my valued reader. You can surely imagine that it is not easy to establish yourself as a new and unknown author. The time and effort an author spends on his books has a lot to do with idealism and, of course, the joy of writing. Applause is the bread of the artist, this saying also applies to authors. Our applause is made up of stars, recommendations and (hopefully good) reviews.

If you liked this book, I would be very pleased if you would reward me with a corresponding rating, a recommendation and maybe even a small review. Thanks a lot for that!

All the best for you and your bacteria friends!

Bibliography

[1] Y. N. Harari, Eine kurze Geschichte der Menschheit, 2015.

[2] L. N. R. Fund, „Study finds eating fiber prevents gut bacteria from eating you," 11 2016. [Online]. Available: https://www.fnr.lu/research-with-impact-fnr-highlight/eating-fiber-prevents-gut-bacteria-eating-you/. [Accessed 1 11 2019].

[3] E. Mayer, „Das Verdauungssystem als Supercomputer," in *Das zweite Gehirn*, p. 19.

[4] E. Mayer, „Der Darm als Sinnesorgan," in *Das zweite Gehirn*, p. 66.

[5] E. Mayer, „Ungesunde Erinnerungen - die Wirkung frühkindlicher Erfahrungen auf den Dialog zwischen Darm und Gehirn," in *Das zweite Gehirn*, p. 109.

[6] E. Mayer, „Emotionen in neuem Licht," in *Das zweite Gehirn*, p. 139.

[7]   „https://www.bundesgesundheitsministerium.de/,“ Bundesministerium für Gesundheit, [Online]. Available: https://www.bundesgesundheitsministerium.de/themen/praevention/gesundheitsgefahren/depression.html.

[8]   „https://www.spektrum.de,“ Spektrum der Wissenschaft Verlagsgesellschaft mbH, [Online]. Available: https://www.spektrum.de/news/ist-glueck-eine-frage-der-gene/1301430.

[9]   „myFairtrade,“ Fair Trade Handels AG, [Online]. Available: https://www.myfairtrade.com/gesundheit/. [Zugriff am 11 2019].

[10] M. Pollan, Lebens-Mittel: Eine Verteidigung gegen die industrielle Nahrung und den Diätenwahn, 2009.

[11] F. T. H. AG, „myfairtrade,“ Fair Trade Handels AG, [Online]. Available: https://www.myfairtrade.com/weizengrassaft-pulver.html.

[12] E. Mayer, „Der Darm unter Verdacht,“ in *Das zweite Gehirn*, p. 86 ff..

[13] F. T. H. AG, „myfairtrade,“ Fair Trade Handels AG, [Online]. Available: https://www.myfairtrade.com/gesundheit/verdauung/bentonit/.

[14] „www.naehrwertrechner.de,“ Stefanie C. Poplutz, [Online]. Available:

https://www.naehrwertrechner.de/naehrwerte/Weizen+Voll
korn/. [Accessed 2019].

[15] W. Bartens, „Entschlackung? Es gibt kein Abfluss-Frei für den
Körper," in *Schluss mit den falschen Vorschriften*, p. Pos.450.

[16] N. N. Taleb, in *Antifragilität: Anleitung für eine Welt, die wir
nicht verstehen*, p. 162.

[17] „https://www.klartext-nahrungsergaenzung.de/,"
Verbraucherzentrale NRW e.V., 2017. [Online]. Available:
https://www.klartext-
nahrungsergaenzung.de/wissen/projekt-klartext-
nahrungsergaenzung/informationen/rechtliches/allgemeine-
rechtliche-aspekte-zu-nahrungsergaenzungsmitteln-13248.
[Accessed 01 11 2019].

[18] „https://gutepillen-schlechtepillen.de/," Gute Pillen -
Schlechte Pillen - Gemeinnützige Gesellschaft für
unabhängige Gesundheitsinformation mbH, [Online].
Available: https://gutepillen-schlechtepillen.de/. [Zugriff am
1 11 2019].

[19] I. Ben-Barak, „Fortpflanzen, fortpflanzen, fortpflanzen," in
Kleine Wunderwerke, p. 16.

[20] E. Mayer, „Kann eine Ernährungsumstellung die
Darmmikrobiota verändern?," in *Das zweite Gehirn*, p. 214.

[21] K. Zahnweh, „mikrobiominfo," Katrin Zahnweh, [Online].
Available:

https://mikrobiominfo.de/gesund/schwangerschaft. [Zugriff
am 1 11 2019].

[22] „spektrum.de," Spektrum der Wissenschaft
Verlagsgesellschaft mbH, [Online]. Available:
https://www.spektrum.de/wissen/die-fuenf-grossen-fragen-
der-gluecksforschung/1404493.

[23] M. Pollan, Essen Sie nichts, was Ihre Großmutter nicht als
Essen erkannt hätte.

[24] „www.bvl.bund.de," Bundesamt für Verbraucherschutz und
Lebensmittelsicherheit (BVL), [Online]. Available:
https://www.bvl.bund.de/DE/01_Lebensmittel/04_Antragste
llerUnternehmen/04_Zusatzstoffe/lm_zusatzstoffe_Zulassun
g_node.html. [Zugriff am 01 11 2019].

[25] „https://www.nature.com/," [Online]. Available:
https://www.nature.com/articles/nature14232.epdf?referrer
_access_token=HxLQjdYRNAcZfzFwx-
r84tRgN0jAjWel9jnR3ZoTv0NbBDjcTUxE_5DwCAU7G8vbLDW
pEOi11ft-
sNe96llKrqB5q4HQKkKCcaeHNg_SnTHiRLrQ096jrDCEigmNb9s
l0a2iAiCLlytleZNor3SelFN-
weCErGPClx94mrKHlcqXtveXq9lwkv_U. [Zugriff am 01 11
2019].

[26] E. Mayer, „Darmmikroben und die Gefahren der modernen
Ernährung," in *Das zweite Gehirn*, p. 244.

[27] C. Schöps, „www.zeit.de,“ [Online]. Available:
       https://www.zeit.de/2019/22/fette-fettzellen-fettsaeuren-
       omega-3-giulia-enders. [Accessed 01 11 2019].

[28] N. B. D. S. Codeathon, „https://www.ncbi.nlm.nih.gov,“
       [Online]. Available:
       https://www.ncbi.nlm.nih.gov/pmc/articles/PMC6529202/.
       [Accessed 01 11 2019].

[29] „scinexx.de,“ [Online]. Available:
       https://www.scinexx.de/news/medizin/verraet-die-
       mundflora-spaeteres-uebergewicht/. [Zugriff am 01 11 2019].

[30] „foodwatch.org,“ foodwatch Deutschland, [Online].
       Available:
       https://www.foodwatch.org/de/informieren/werbeluegen/pr
       odukte/verbesserung-vorgetaeuscht/danone-activia/?L=0.
       [Accessed 01 11 2019].